Contents

Acknowledgements

I would like to thank all my work colleagues for putting up with me while I completed this study. I would also like to thank all service users and carers who, with managers and field workers, enthusiastically gave me their time, both as interviewees and in planning this research.

This work is a completely revised version of a dissertation towards the award of MSc in Policy Studies at Bristol University School for Advanced Urban Studies and I would also like to thank Marilyn Taylor, my dissertation supervisor, for her support. I emphasise that this paper is the work of the author, and any conclusions reached are the views of the author and may or may not be shared by the author's employers, Dudley Metropolitan Borough Council Social Services Department. Nevertheless, I hope that locally and nationally it stimulates discussion as to the nature and meaning of 'empowerment'.

I would like to dedicate this work to my mother, Phyllis Servian (1917-1995) who always encouraged me to treat education as a life-long endeavour, and empowered me, in one sense of the word, to undertake the production of this work.

Finally, my thanks also go to Dawn Louise Pudney and Julia Mortimer from The Policy Press, for their commitment in preparing this work for publication.

THEORISING EMPOWERMENT

Individual power and community care

Richard Servian

First published in Great Britain in 1996 by

The Policy Press
University of Bristol
Rodney Lodge
Grange Road
Bristol BS8 4EA

Telephone: (0117) 973 8797
Fax: (0117) 973 7308
E-mail: tpp@bris.ac.uk

ISBN 1 86134 006 0

Richard Servian is the Service Manager (Resources for children with disabilities) at Dudley Social Services.

The Policy Press works to counter discrimination on grounds of gender, race, disability, age and sexuality.

Printed in Great Britain by Bourne Press Limited.

Abstract

This study explores individual perceptions of power, focusing on health and social services for people with learning disabilities in one metropolitan borough. It starts by investigating what empowerment is, and goes on to question attempts to empower carers and users through organisational and structural change. Concentrating on recent decentralisation and market initiatives, it asserts that one reason why such models may fail is because of their rationalist basis, which does not include a substantial model of individual behaviour, and so excludes an understanding of how individuals are empowered or disempowered. Policy studies are also criticised for not generally including a psychological dimension.

This qualitative study has been designed to compare the perceptions that carers, users, workers and managers have, of historical and present power structures within learning disability services. The study brings together a theoretical framework from a number of disciplines in order to analyse how the individual perceives power. These areas include the sociological and the strategic, but the emphasis is on the psychological. Tajfel's (1981) Social Identity Theory sees individuals choosing between individual and group approaches in developing a positive social identity, and this theory is used to help analyse the approaches individuals take in using health and social services to seek empowerment. Seligman's (1975) theory of 'learned helplessness' uses behaviour theory to identify the cognitive and behavioural causes of depression. It is used here to help identify the circumstances under which people feel disempowered.

The findings show a picture of contradictions and tensions in power relations between carers, users, workers and managers. A suggestion is, that despite policy changes, historical power relations are reproducing themselves and users continue to be disempowered. Some of the basic causes of individual disempowerment continue to operate.

Finally, it is suggested that the framework of analysis used here could be used positively to help avoid disempowerment, to better inform policy development, and to show how individuals can participate effectively in policy making and implementation.

Introduction

There is a basic contradiction about empowerment in many studies. The assumption is made here that when we talk about empowerment we are talking about empowering the individual. Yet dominant methods and proposals for empowerment have tended to emphasise structural and organisational processes, with the individual in the position of a manipulated element rather than necessarily the important part of the process. What is missing is the view of the individual and an analysis of how an individual can be empowered or disempowered. Of course the assumption of a shared value of individual empowerment may be quite fallacious, and what the empowerment project may really be about is increasing the power of certain 'helping' organisations, or some other notion of empowerment – this, too, is not clear.

Not only is the personal analysis and implementation of empowerment missing, but there is actually little agreement between professionals and users as to what this means, and how different people understand and experience power and empowerment.

The 'Personal is Political' was a feminist slogan of the seventies, and reflected frustration with the failure to see individuals as key actors of politics, and political analyses, which rather seemed to see people as a large undifferentiated mass. A concern here is that such issues have not reached the consciousness of either policy makers or theoreticians in the area of community care or of empowerment, and there is an urgent need to recognise the validity of the slogan, and to ask why it has been ignored. The attempt here is to bring individuals back into the policy process, but also to analyse from the individual's perspective why this is so difficult. This report also looks at whether there is concensus that individuals, particularly at the receiving end of public policy practice, are to be the main beneficiaries of processes meant to lead to empowerment.

These questions are explored by analysing perceptions of power by community care participants themselves. This is done by drawing a framework from different theoretical analyses: broadly, the structural, the strategic and the psychological. While believing this study is relevant to all situations where disempowerment is an issue, there is a focus here on two groups that have particularly suffered from a lack of power: people with learning disabilities and their carers. Perceptions of power positions of professionals and managers in health and social services' provision for people with learning disabilities are also looked at.

There have been many changes to services for people with learning disabilities in approximately the last 20 years. National policies have moved from an emphasis on large institutions to an emphasis on community support particularly by way of joint health and social services learning disability teams, to the present emphasis on market analogies. Such changes reflect what is happening elsewhere in public services with decentralisation strategies and market structures. Both have had at least a political promise of empowerment. The impact such changes have had on the perception of empowerment by carers and users, and on the exercise of power by professionals and managers is questioned here.

> ... who makes decisions for me? Who is preventing me from doing this and telling me to do that? Who is programming my movements and activities? Who is forcing me to live in a particular place when I work in another? How are these decisions on which my life is completely articulated taken? All these questions seem to be fundamental ones today. And I don't believe that the question of 'who exercises power?' can be resolved unless that other question 'how does it happen?' is resolved .... (Foucault, 1984, p 103)

This study does not pretend to do more than begin to answer Foucault's questions, nor does it use Foucault's historical analysis. The emphasis is on similar individual concerns and the impact on individuals of the structural framework.

A general presumption behind ideas of empowerment in the area of this study appears to be that people with learning disabilities are powerless. Is this true, in their and their carers perceptions? If it is, why is there a feeling of powerlessness? What steps can be taken to change this situation? Do front-line workers and managers perceive themselves as having the means to empower? Or is their power, in effect, used against rather than for users and carers?

This study is also about the individual and the policy process. It is not possible to talk about influencing policy without talking about individual perceptions of power and who has power to enable change. A definition of 'having power' may be 'influencing policy', and a measure of the value of this study will be how far it helps individuals who perceive themselves as powerless to influence policy at some level that means positive change for them. In looking at power from an individual's perspective we are looking at how individuals can influence policy and how political processes can be made more sensitive to individual influence. This issue is not going to be looked at from the starting point of policy theory, which generally ignores the individual. Rather, it is the author's intention to address the question of individual power from theories that emphasise the individual's perspective.

Within this study the author intends looking at 'power' from a number of theoretical positions and tries to draw a framework that can enable an analysis of perceptions of power by different participants. In Chapter 1 the author explores some of the difficulties in defining empowerment and then sets the political background to this study, looking at some of the 'grand plans' that presently purport to lead to empowerment. He questions whether such strategic and structural solutions really can live up to their promise of empowerment, if indeed that is their aim, and suggests that they lack a substantial theory of personal behaviour.

Chapter 2 presents some basic theoretical perspectives that are used to help define power as far as participants in public services are concerned, and to provide the basis for the interview schedule for the qualitative study. The author has chosen approaches to help define power as it affects users of public services, adding psychological and individual definitions to the structural and strategic solutions of the market/state/citizenship debate. Chapter 3 provides a practical backdrop to the study itself, with a discussion of some of the existing analyses of power within services for people with learning disabilities. The author also goes on to discuss the methodology of the qualitative study used here, summarising and attempting to analyse the responses of interviewees. Chapter 4 presents some conclusions and ways forward. A suggested use of the findings is to form an audit structure that could be used to check how user-oriented policies and services are.

Chapter 1

Empowerment and reason

In this chapter the author initially concentrates on looking at what empowerment is and who is to be empowered. It is suggested that this is not as clear as it may seem, as there is little agreement about what power is and how it operates, while empowerment has different meanings in different contexts. Empowerment is something so essential that it is not just sought by those who are objectively perceived as powerless. It is sought by people at all levels for differing reasons. It is a concept now used by employers to maximise returns from their workforce, while the interest in empowerment by official organisations, such as the Audit Commission, mean that there are now official definitions of who is to be empowered, in effect, to ration resources.

From the various ways the term empowerment has been used, the author proposes a working definition of what empowerment is and goes on to argue that the many strategic and structural policies behind public services have failed to empower vulnerable individuals. The problem arises from a rationalist approach including a belief that organisational change is all that is needed. The individual has been forgotten and there is a theoretical need to add wider psychological perspectives to those presently implicit. Where such perspectives already exist they are incomplete or questionable.

As examples, the author looks at a political strategy and a structure that have both been declared as being about empowerment and questions whether they really are. The author looks at:

- Decentralisation: this has been seen as a major strategy for empowerment, particularly by Labour councils. It is a set of administrative devices rather than an ideological structure, but it has been proposed as an alternative to the structural changes of the market. The author suggests that in reality it is about the defence of local government through improved administration, and it reflects a 'rationalist' approach that includes a belief in the scientific basis of government, but not an explicit model of individual behaviour which, it is suggested, is essential to understand empowerment and disempowerment.

- Markets: structural changes to public services by way of market systems are now advocated by left (through market socialism) and right as empowering. The author suggests that the psychological mechanism of 'self-interest' behind such changes is too narrow and the reality again is administrative changes rather than empowerment.

It is suggested that the reason why structures and strategies do not appear to empower is because such rationalist approaches forget the individual, and are based on an inadequate analysis of human behaviour.

What is empowerment?

Over the last ten years or so, the use of the terms 'power' and 'empowerment' have become common, and are included in discussions on both the British government's community care policy and in the description of the position of disabled people in society. These terms are rarely defined by those people that use them. Rather, it is presumed we all know what is meant by power and empowerment. The author will discuss here whether there is any general agreement as to the use of either concept or whether different participants have different interpretations of these issues.

What do we mean by empowerment?

This is not a straightforward question, as we first need to define 'power', and to theorise what power is and how it affects people, in order to understand what happens when people have or do not have power. Such theorising is attempted in the next chapter, although as we shall see, this is more easily said than done. Power is a contested concept that is continually being redefined, and this work continues that process.

In seeking a working definition for 'empowerment' there are equal problems as this term has different meanings to different people. Different notions of empowerment have been used by different groups at all levels of status or class. The following are samples of these different viewpoints with brief examples of those proposing change. The term 'empowerment' is not necessarily used by stakeholders in all these samples, but it is suggested that they are all about empowerment.

- **Empowerment as control of industry.** Industry has historically been the battleground for competing claims for empowerment between employers and organised labour, although both groups may be seen as having resources presently denied to many disabled people. Until recently, the British Labour Party Constitution proposed "to secure for the workers by hand or by brain the full fruits of their industry ...". In the eighties a frequent clarion call for employers was for "their right to manage ...".

- **Empowerment as changing workplace technology.** Pascale (1990) has reported how the term 'empowerment' is used by Honda in Japan to develop a high quality workforce, with the overriding motivation of increasing company profit. Empowerment in this view represents a different form of organisation in the workplace from that produced by the scientific management approach. A specific role on the production line or in the office is replaced with a more flexible view of the skills of the worker and of their ability to take on a wider number of roles. While share ownership may come into this, empowerment here is not generally about worker control and management. A question here is whether empowerment in the community care context is also more about the technology of providing a service rather than a say in the control of an organisation.

- **Empowerment as access to democratic processes.** The right to vote, or a say in some other way in political policies, is a major campaign by a large number of people throughout the world. The South African elections in 1994 were the result of campaigning by many. In Britain there is still a struggle for people with a history of institutional care to obtain the vote.

- **Empowerment as taking leadership.** Political leaders, senior managers and club and society committees are frequently the centre of competition for leadership. In recent years, in a number of national organisations for disabled people, there has been competition for senior positions between disabled and non-disabled people. Empowerment in this context is about the powerless taking the leadership of an organisation to obtain power.

- **Empowerment as changing the value base of an institution.** Hilary Rose (1994) asserted the need for feminist science and research as a response to a paternalist science and technology seen as historically essential to world domination and imperialism. There are similar questions raised about the traditional role of health and social services professionals in dominating the lives of disabled people, and the need for a change of philosophy (Barnes, 1991).

- **Empowerment as meeting specific needs or rationing resources.** In implementing community care legislation, the Audit Commission (1992a) talk of empowering users and carers, while emphasising the need for eligibility criteria. Empowerment of users and carers in this notion is seen as taking place through the development of market systems to give greater choice in meeting the individual needs of a selected few. Empowerment also features through the involvement of users and carers in planning, effectively participating in the rationing of the service. This view of empowerment is looked at in more detail later.

- **Empowerment as permission.** Empowering your bank to invest your money, or empowering a member of staff to work in a particular, agreed way are examples of this definition. Empowerment is limited to a specific action or group of actions, for which permission is given by a manager or another individual who has power over those actions. If service users are empowered, is it only in terms of permission in very restricted circumstances?

- **Empowerment as freeing from government.** National Empowerment Television in the USA is a right-wing station committed to freeing people from 'big' government. From a different perspective, empowerment has also been used to describe the freedom felt by young people in the sixties in rebelling against authority (Neville, 1995). Policies of decentralisation may also come under this heading.

- **Empowerment as advocacy.** We all have the potential, but we all need support to get what we want or need. The provision of advocacy helps us get there. Solicitors, brokers, citizen advocates, and parents or friends may empower in this way.

- **Empowerment as spiritual enlightenment.** Most religions and certain philosophies tend to promote empowerment through spiritual rather than material fulfilment. Sogyal Rinpoche (1992) describes the room of his buddhist teacher as "the room of empowerment".

There is an interesting discussion to be had in contrasting these and other interpretations, but for the purposes of this paper they are presented in order to explore similarities and not differences, to ask whether there is a common thread between views of what empowerment is. None of these positions solely emphasise the focus of this study – the empowerment of disabled people or those in relatively low power positions. In a real way they represent attempts by individuals at all power levels to meet certain needs. Within all of these definitions there are individuals or groups attempting to promote change in ways that potentially fulfil certain of the individuals involved, although this may be in a very limited way. Even in the most restricted views of empowerment, such as 'empowerment as permission', the individuals given permission may see themselves as benefiting from that action.

Despite the doubts about what power is, the author suggests that this common denominator is enough to form a relatively crude working definition of empowerment for this study, that through having power individuals can at least partly meet their own 'needs'. If they have been able to follow their own interests, to feel fulfilment or to meet their own material needs, an assumption is that they have displayed their own power in doing so – they are empowered.

This means that 'empowerment' and 'needs' are perceived here as being interrelated. If this is the case, the first question is, which needs must be met for people to be perceived as empowered? There is a long history of debate as to what 'needs' are and whether they all can or should be met (see, eg, Bradshaw, 1972). It is presumed here that the reader knows about that debate despite Peter Taylor-Goodby's (1991) assertion that there appears to be little agreement among theoreticians that there can be any reliable definitions of need, let alone agreement. A problem may be that participants in the debate may be arguing about different issues. It is not clear that the aim of the debate is always to meet needs or to empower.

Doyal and Gough (1991) attempted to define needs from the 'first principles' of human life and in terms of which philosophies and strategies needed to be followed to most fully meet needs. They suggested that two basic needs, of autonomy and survival, were the preconceptions for the achieving of other goals. 'Human liberation' represented the optimisation of needs and this was achieved through the continual overcoming of boundaries and maximising creativity. This notion of the essential importance of personal autonomy is shared with psychoanalytic theory.

So if needs and empowerment are related, then, from this analysis, 'empowerment' may be best seen as 'moves toward autonomy'. A problem in using such a definition in practice, in helping, for instance, a local social services department define it's role, is that the practical need to define 'needs' may be more to do with organisational demands to ration resources than helping an individual to become autonomous. If empowerment and needs are related concepts then empowerment, like certain definitions of need, may become a method of rationing scarce resources.

Official empowerment

> The first aim (of the community care legislation) is to empower the service users and their carers ... (Audit Commission, 1992a)

The Audit Commision do not identify which users and carers are to be empowered, but indicate that this is the role of social services departments. This means that there will be, in each area, an official view of who is to be empowered.

If empowerment is about individuals meeting their own needs, then any narrowing down of the concept will be disempowering. If 'need' has been continually redefined to ration budgets, then so long as an official view of empowerment also means access to resources, we can expect this too to be continually redefined, to restrict who is to be empowered and by how much. In this, and other ways, empowerment is a living word, whose meaning is changing or becoming distorted.

Is any project of empowerment subject to those with the power to redefine the concept? This raises the question of whether official intervention, (for example, direct funding or social services resources), is the key to empowerment, and whether the Audit Commission are correct in believing that empowerment can come through legislation that is essentially about the allocation of resources. Certainly in a capitalist society, money is a key to improving living standards, whether this is spent directly by service users or on their behalf by professionals. If needs are seen only in material terms, then, as the author starts from the assertion of a link between the two concepts, empowerment must be achievable through financial means.

This rationalist view of empowerment and self-worth ignores the community, spiritual and feeling side to humanity, access to which is also, according to Doyal and Gough, a key to autonomy. This alternative perspective includes democratic rights – to involvement by individual citizens in decision making and other participative processes, and the values these rights represent. It is questionable whether these are central to official views of empowerment centred on resource rationing, as in community care policies.

The mechanical or rationalist view of human behaviour displayed in official views of empowerment is reflected in behavioural theories that see people as only responding to material concerns. This position has become incorporated into policies said to be about empowerment, as will be discussed later. It is argued that the rationalist view makes it easier for individual need and empowerment to be devalued because of a limited conception of power and behaviour generalised across groups. If it is empowerment of individual users of services that we wish to address then we need to look at power and empowerment as felt by the individual. This paper attempts to address the gap in theory in this area.

Who is to be empowered?

The British Council of Organisations of Disabled People (BCODP) believes that an analysis of power relations is central to an understanding of the position of disabled people in British society. Colin Barnes (1991) talks of:

> ... a proliferation of professional helpers who exercise considerable power over those they profess to be helping ... disabled people's ability to participate in the economic and social life of the community is frequently adversely affected by this provision.

This and similar analyses have begun to have an impact on social care practice. The ABCD pack on training workers to deal with abuse of disabled children (NSPCC, 1994) declares:

> Philosophy: That children and adults with impairments are dis-abled by the way that society is structured; that abuse is a misuse of power ....

Professionals and carers are seen as tending to reinforce the powerlessness of disabled people. One response is to support professionals and carers, through training, in understanding such individual relationships and redefining their roles.

The notion that individual professionals can empower by changing their practice presumes that those professionals share a view of empowerment with disabled people. It also presumes that professionals can substantially change what they do even if the organisation they work for, or the political policies they work under, do not change in the same direction. Such a position would seem to counter the notion that power relations dominate. This difficulty is recognised in the BCODP's advocacy of civil rights legislation as tackling power issues in a wider political context than the individual professional–disabled person relationship.

It is not clear that direct empowerment of disabled people need be the only possible outcome of the BCODP's analysis of power relations. Although their proposed response is different, the analysis of the American radical right has similarities to that of the BCODP. They also argue that the welfare state is paternalistic and anti-libertarian.

Whereas the BCODP argue for a shift in resources, Atherton (1989) reports the view of the radical right, that any state that has the power to shift resources from one group to another represents a form of economic tyranny. The right's response is to focus on the re-empowerment of those 'coerced' into funding the poor.

This position has become essential to the view of the right in government internationally, and the condition of the poor (if this is a concern at all) is seen as only developed through the enhancement of the wealth of those individuals already with resources. An example of this is the British Government's refusal in 1993 and 1994 to support a civil rights bill for disabled people largely on the grounds of cost to business, and the argument that the future lay in businesses' ability to offer employment and not rights.

Are the radical right alone in seeing the empowerment project as not being about the direct empowerment of disabled people and users of services, but on 'liberating' the already powerful?

A large proportion of our earlier list of different notions of empowerment were as much about giving power to already powerful groups as to the powerless. Advocacy is more available to those who can afford to pay solicitors, while shareholders benefit from changing workplace technology. Managers, rather than social services users, may be empowered as rationers of resources.

While empowerment may be a new word, the project of empowerment is very old and may be essential to human need, as Doyal and Gough (1991) suggest. The argument here is that power is an essential concept for all individuals and power relations affect all participants in a power network. This means that a project of empowerment could, in reality, affect any individual in any part of the power web. It should not be presumed that an empowerment project is *automatically* about, for example, empowering social services users. If traditional power relations dominate, as Foucault (1979a) argues, then the empowerment of the more powerful may be more likely. Hence, some notions of empowerment could be methods by which exploitation can also take place, as perhaps with the Honda example earlier, or lead to little change of those with power. Democratic processes may leave the same groups of people in government as before democracy. In the British parliament able white men dominate as they did before universal franchise.

If it cannot be automatically guaranteed who the person or group to be empowered is, then if empowerment of the powerless is the issue, this cannot be left to structures designed to empower, or organisations constituted so as to empower. One type of organisation from this point of view can be little more empowering than any other organisation, as far as many individuals are concerned. If empowerment projects are to be focused, a theoretical perspective is needed in which individual empowerment can be understood, and that is a project of this paper.

Empowerment and structures

If we assume 'empowerment' is about giving power to or meeting the needs of those with less power, then much of the political history of the twentieth century in Britain has been about empowerment – from the moves to universal franchise, the development of the Labour Party and the social democratic dream of using the capitalist creation of wealth for the benefit of all; to the development of the welfare state and anti-discrimination laws; and to the more recent moves of public sector decentralisation and attempts to democratise the marketplace. While many such grand plans have successfully implanted some notion of empowerment there continue to be many, particularly the more vulnerable, who do not appear to benefit. Two reasons are suggested. Firstly, some of the moves theoretically empower, but in reality become predominantly administrative changes. It is assumed here that politicians are genuine in seeking empowerment for those less powerful than themselves through such changes, and a result that fails to empower is not always deliberate. Secondly, too little regard is given to the perception of power in as far as the individual is concerned, because of the emphasis and belief in grand plans, and the associated mechanical and behaviourist conception of human behaviour.

Behind the grand plans are ideological perspectives more based on traditional structures, and economic rather than democratic forces, and the power inherent in those. Foucault (1979b) sees such creeds as aspects of 'rationality' or the dominant view of the world based on Hobbesian reason, rather than any natural tendency. Rationality, in this view, is a tool of governance that legitimates political systems and power structures, through encouraging a belief that such systems have a scientific and hence correct basis.

The problems of grand political theory are illustrated by concentrating on the most recent changes mentioned above – 'decentralisation' and 'market' approaches, which have been influential philosophies in local government changes in the last 10 years. While decentralisation is an administrative device and the market an ideological structure, both have been presented as being about empowerment of public service users.

Decentralisation for whom?

Decentralisation is a strategy rather than a new structure, but it is widely seen as a method of improving the responsiveness of local government and health services, and carrying the possibility of improving state services without market initiatives (eg, Hambleton and Hoggett, 1990).

Broadly speaking, decentralisation is seen as empowering because of the closer relationships between residents and officials that is said to be an aspect of more local services, but also because of involvement of residents in democratic processes, such as council committees. Decentralisation was a major local government (and health authorities) project of the eighties. One reason for an interest in decentralisation in the eighties was the defence of local government, in the context of the Conservative national government's tendency to centralise decision making, and its attack on Labour local government. Decentralisation became a major initiative, particularly by Labour councils, although not exclusively so. Empowerment of local residents appears to have been a relatively minor aim in practice, although may sometimes have been a consequence.

Hambleton (1988) identified that decentralisation can be achieved to different extents, from the purely managerial to substantial democracy, and for different objectives – from democratic accountability to managerial control, and to public relations. This leads to the question of whether decentralisation, when used in practice, is about managerial effectiveness or user responsiveness.

Challis (1990) has highlighted the mixed uses and results of decentralisation in social services departments, and argues that, in many cases, change is only partial, with an underlying desire not to disrupt services, and widespread scepticism among front-line workers that decentralisation is to the benefit of users. Beresford and Croft (1986) reinforce such scepticism in their study of patch social work in East Sussex in which they see little power to service users, despite the more local nature of organisation.

Conservative national government in the eighties criticised Labour local government for financial mismanagement, and the greater emphasis on audit, such as through the Audit Commision, was a tool of such criticism, although it also represented an ideological change of emphasis, to be measured by cost rather than service. Decentralisation in local government can be seen as a response to this, an attempt to defend local government through the introduction of processes that emphasise greater managerial controls with at least a façade of more accessible services. Community care policy has been no exception to this with considerable interest from the Audit Commision (1992a, b) and the emphasis on cost, process and more narrow priorities rather than the practice of meeting a wider number and variety of needs. Far from giving power, a major area of interest in decentralisation is to achieve stronger power at the centre.

While in many of its definitions decentralisation can be seen as providing at least a basis of empowering public service users, it provides no explicit model of human behaviour. In providing a strategy, and a political assertion of empowerment, a presumption appears to be of automatic exploitation by users of such a strategy. In so far as behaviour is analysed it is implicit, and it is something about distance of officials from users rather than a practical analysis of individual involvement.

This model of state organisation has its roots in rationalism, which, according to Foucault (1979b), is basic to all models of government around the notion of the state, with reason having replaced violence as an instrument of power. Within the perception of rationality is the support for objective scientific versions of reality, whether or not this objectivity is real rather than emanating from the interests of the powerful. Basic to this is the belief that dominant political systems and strategies are rational and legitimate, whether or not they are fully based on substantial theory. Similarly there appears to be no substantial behavioural theory inherent in decentralisation strategies, although the mechanism of decentralisation appears scientific.

The care market

With the April 1993 community care changes, services – whether decentralised or traditionally provided – now have a different model of operation, based on the market. Market systems are based on a more explicit view of human behaviour, as will be discussed later.

The introduction of this model attracted no substantial party political criticism, although the lack of funding has done so since. This was despite criticism of similar market models in the health service both prior to and since implementation, and despite deeper 'privatisation' inherent in the community care changes, as compared with the concurrent health changes. Does this suggest a widespread acceptance of market models and implicit criticisms of decentralisation initiatives? If so, this may be less to do with a belief in empowerment through the market, than with the promise to local government of a lead role in community care and money to go with it. If decentralisation in practice was largely about defending local government, then the market in community care appears to be so too, and a more defensible one, despite the majority of councils' different political perspectives.

The model of community care now in operation is based on the new right's public choice models of government, and based on self-interest. Like decentralisation, and despite assertions of the Audit Commision and others, the changes are not intrinsically empowering.

Rather, the reality is that the market changes are really based on political, administrative and economic needs than the needs of social services users. In so far as the market is about empowerment, the author suggests that it is based on an incomplete view of human behaviour.

Public choice

Public choice theories (eg, Buchanan, 1978) that lie behind market models of government developed around criticisms of the efficiency of public servants. They make 'self-interest' a core value and a method of analysis. This endeavour is not exclusive to public choice theoreticians. Barry (1990) asserts that one of the major arguments for the market is that the exchange system driven by self-interest will accidentally maximise welfare more effectively than purposeful intervention.

Public choice theory takes this a step further and presumes a strong psychological mechanism based on self-interest for all behaviour. Such an analysis of the behaviour of civil servants (Niskanen, 1973) was very influential on Nicholas Ridley, who wrote the Niskanen paper foreword and was the architect of the 1988 and 1989 Local Government Acts that brought market systems to councils. In this paper, the behaviour of 'senior bureaucrats' is criticised as being based on self-interest with the aims of building empires and budget maximisation. Niskanen's response is to suggest that public bureaucracies could be reformulated to make self-interest congruent with policy interests.

Community care is perhaps the latest public policy to draw on the market solutions that public choice advocates see as crucial to public sector reform. It introduces a 'quasi-market' (LeGrand, 1990), rather than a full market, in that service users are not purchasing services directly. A local government officer (the care manager) purchases such services from a market of public and private providers, based on an assessment of the user. The 'bureaucracy' is thus converted into a system based on market mechanisms.

From the public choice perspective, the role of the social care professional as a budget controller, effectively the role of care manager, makes the self-interest of the professional more congruent with budget control where this is in the interest of the organisation, than with meeting the needs of users. Given government cuts, the consequent financial difficulties of councils and the role of the Audit Commission, budget control may well be the priority and the reason for the changes. In the context of budgeting priorities, such a self-interest model does not appear to centre on empowerment of users, who are not central players in purchasing their own care, but on administration.

Public choice theories differ from mass sociological theory in postulating psychological mechanisms for choice, but it is not clear that self-interest is a main psychological mechanism. Even if self-interest is the key, it is far from certain that non-market results are as far removed from the public interest as Niskanen suggests. Some civil servants' self-interest may lie in reducing stress by appropriately serving the public, or policy interests, without market inducements. Nor is it clear that self-interest solutions create more effective bureaucracies, rather than being divisive and less accountable, particularly if the link with democratic processes is broken, as public choice protagonists propose. Competition between providers may improve costs but not necessarily empower.

As with decentralisation, a rational view of human behaviour dominates. The notion of humans mechanically responding to simple notions of rewards and interests is prevalent in self-interest perspectives. Clegg (1989) historically traces this behavioural and intentional view of human behaviour, to Hobbes and the development of the state in terms of rationality rather than violence, but:

> In some respects the evacuation of the classical liberal concern with the specificity of the person has left behavioural political science with little other than the shell of the traditional conception. The shell consisted in a certain metaphoricality in which mechanistic, atomistic and above all, causal images reigned supreme. (Clegg, 1989, p 42)

The notion of 'behavioural political science' itself reinforces the notion of a rational basis to market or other structures in politics and the public service, despite the lack of a substantial model of individual behaviour within at least the public choice version of such science.

To summarise the argument here, the great structural, strategic and political proposals on public services appear to have in common the promise of empowerment but the danger of being mere administrative changes. Such dangers appear to stem from a reliance on grand solutions and the associated rationalist position, rather than looking at the individual. They have in common a poverty in their analysis of individual behaviour. Public choice models do explicitly address the psychological dimension, through 'self-interest'. However, this is narrowly based, also on the rationalist perspective and an incomplete mechanical model of human behaviour.

The problems of defining structures for empowerment are complicated by the difficulties outlined earlier, of defining what we mean by empowerment and who is to be empowered. It is suggested here that we must take a wider view to begin to understand the individual basis of power and to comprehend how individuals perceive power and powerlessness. Structural and strategic theories tell us little about how power is perceived and how it affects individuals. Rather, the tendency is to see individuals as indefensible victims or automatons to be trampled over by great machines. But is there any point in encouraging an individual perspective on empowerment if structures cannot deliver? It is exactly because of the failure of structures and strategies to respond to individual needs that analysis of individual perspectives on power needs to be made, so that existing structures can be challenged.

Foucault (1983) also challenges the notion of political grand plans, advocating the study of power strategies and the discourse historically by which power structures are achieved, of what historically and presently lies behind relations of power. Such power relations are not seen as being about a single dominant power but about a variety of relations around individuals and institutions. This study, while not following Foucaultian methods of historical or 'genealogical' analysis, attempts to analyse such power relations from the perceptions of participants.

Chapter 2

The personal is political

If we are concerned about individual empowerment then we need to be concerned about the role of individuals in policy, and in the context of this study, health and social services users and carers in particular. We must be concerned not only about what happens to individuals in developing their view and assumptions about politics, but also what processes arise that lead to involvement or non-involvement in 'political' processes. How do outside power, policy and actions impact on such processes? This, it is suggested, means looking for new theoretical approaches to add to the predominant analyses in policy theory that tend to emphasise macro views by way of politics, sociology and organisational analyses.

The theoretical approaches presented in this chapter are not meant as a complete world view nor a grand plan for policy analysis. In Harré's (1993) terms the author is not trying to set inalienable rules either, rather he is presenting a set of analogies. The attempt is to bring together various perspectives to link the individual's interpretation and construction of the world, with the influence of wider power structures and strategies that may be defined by policy initiatives and individuals, or groups, to show such power as people have or make, or are victims of.

Central to such a perspective are psychological analyses of how individuals operate. The theories that are looked at have a base in the scientific rationality that was criticised in Chapter 1, but the substance of the criticisms is not necessarily rationality in itself, but the narrowness in the perception of individual behaviour in politics and policies that it has brought with it.

The choice of psychology theory to use is a difficult one as this area of endeavour is divided between perspectives. Psychodynamic approaches continue to be divided from experimental and behavioural approaches, while experimental approaches divide between those who see cognitive processes as important and those who see human behaviour as explicable through wholly observable behavioural analyses. It is not the author's intention to join this argument here, although he does refer to some of the issues later in the chapter. The author has already suggested the importance of the psychodynamic perspective in the analysis of the importance of 'autonomy' that he sees the notion of empowerment as part of. In choosing the theories here he has tried to find usable theories that can help identify in an observable way what empowerment is and how it may come about, or be denied. The chosen use of theory here does not deny the potency of other theories that are not used. It is suggested here that it is useful to have an approach that does not reinforce differences between subject areas but allies sociological, psychological and other theoretical areas in identifying how power affects the individual.

In this study it is the author's intention to concentrate particularly on two psychological theories: the cognitive behavioural theory of 'learned helplessness' (Seligman, 1975), which he sees as giving a behaviourally defined breakdown of why people feel powerless and do not get involved; and from social psychology – 'social identity theory' (Tajfel, 1981), which is based on studies of groups and presents a view of why people choose to join groups, choose to be identified as members of groups, or choose a more individual approach. From such perspectives the author proposes to obtain some bottom lines for successful involvement of individuals in power processes. The argument here is not that everything is down to the individual: indeed the argument is that what individuals can do is limited by direct, indirect and ideological power structures. Nevertheless, the author also suggests that the psychological level has been much neglected in policy studies. This has become a crucial problem when suddenly we are faced with the problem of attracting citizens or consumers to be involved in public policy, when perhaps the major interest in the past has been how a policy elite can make policy into practice (eg, Hodgwood and Gunn, 1984). The incorporation of psychology analyses into policy enquiry is not new, but it is rare, and nor is it a simple issue. Hilary Graham (1983) saw the separate analyses of policy analysts of caring in material terms, and psychologists in affective terms to have both missed the central points "that caring defines both the identity and the activity of women in western society". Gendered impacts are ignored, but she suggests that such studies could be enabled by bringing perspectives together. An aim of this study is to present a way of looking at power from the individual's viewpoint – the author will attempt to bring together theoretical areas in a way that is practically useful: towards the preparation of a study looking at individuals involved in community care, and their perception of power.

The author contemplates the various levels of analysis using the following theoretical groups of views.

The four faces of power

In order to understand empowerment, and policies and processes that accidentally or purposefully are or are not empowering, we must first understand something about what we mean by power and how it can be interpreted and perceived.

The central emphasis will be on psychology theory and how this can be added to possible strategies available to individuals, but the context of individual action and strategy must be seen within a strict power regime. Power is not seen here purely in terms of direct influence and control, nor is it assumed that we are all merely victims of more powerful forces. However, it is suggested that the individual paths we take, the beliefs we have in our own ability to influence and what choices we do have are severely limited in both our own attributions and in reality.

Lukes' (1974) comparison of three dimensions of power provides a theoretical perspective to the direct, indirect and invisible limitations of power looked at here. He brought together Dahl's conception of power as direct influence, which he saw as just one dimension, with Bachrach and Baratz's (1970) perception of indirect forms of power through a 'mobilisation of bias', which Lukes termed the second dimension. Lukes then added a third 'radical' position, based on Marxian thought, of people being forced by ideology and relations of production to act against their objective interests.

Digeser (1992) takes this analysis to a fourth dimension in looking at the work of Foucault:

> ... insidious, totalising, individuating, disciplinary ... with power operating in structures of thinking and behaviour that previously seemed to be devoid of power relations.

Power is not just, in this analysis, about what people do overtly, covertly or economically to others. It is seen as defining all people who are perceived as social constructions forged by historical power relations.

> It is clear that the kind of enquiry suggested by power[4] differs radically from what seems to flow from the other conceptions of power. Under the first face of power the central question is, 'Who if anyone is exercising power?' Under the second face, 'what issues have been mobilised off the agenda and by whom?' Under the radical conception, 'whose objective interests are being harmed?' Under the fourth face of power the critical issue is 'What kind of subject is being produced?' (Digeser, 1992)

Much of the assertion of Foucault is how power[4] dictates various rules and 'discourses' that govern the social context in which all our economic, political, legal and religious practices are formed. In modern times, 'disciplinary' power has become particularly forged, with the use of school, prison, and hospital to narrow down dispute and exclude difference. The central view is of a suffocating and narrowly defining value system forged by relations of power.

Foucault's analysis of stigmatised views of difference as the result of power relations have been a powerful influence on the women's and gay movements in seeking, instead, to "celebrate the difference". The issues appear to be becoming equally clear for users of social services. Oliver (1990) and the BCODP have reacted to the use of terms such as 'people with disabilities', used by care professionals. The term 'disabled people' is advocated, to encourage disabled people to accept and to be proud of the disability as an essential and important part of the self, rather than an unfortunate and stigmatising add on.

A problem of all four 'faces of power' is an apparent top-down view of power with people tending to be seen as victims, their actions heavily determined by some, mainly invisible outside interest, rather than being seen as active participants, albeit junior partners, in power relations. This reflects the criticisms of psychology that shall be discussed further later, as tending to see people as automatons.

However, the possibility exists of power being used not *against* but *for* people. The exercise of power need not necessarily be oppressive. Indeed, the challenge to oppression can be seen as an object of having power. It can be strongly argued that the role of medical and non-medical professionals is meant in support of people 'in their care'. Obviously, the reality may often be different, but this need not be an inevitability. In any case, in analysing power at all, the possibility is raised of challenging and using it. The answer remains how, and in what circumstances power is used for rather than against, and this may be helped through looking at psychological studies of individuals and at possible generalisations of strategies of protest.

Strategy for individual power: exit, voice, loyalty, neglect?

'Exit', 'voice' and 'loyalty' have been much used recently as symbols of different political and economic stances. The genesis of this symbolic debate was in American corporate life, with Hirschman (1970) seeking to find out why corporate actors could and could not be supported by the public. In Britain the debate has begun to symbolise the difference between neo-liberal models of the market, with exit as the main form of protest where alternative 'purchases' are available; and social democratic ideas of citizenship, where voice is seen as valued. Indeed, Hirschman saw voice as democratic politics itself. Loyalty is seen as a futher response: where people stay in difficult positions through trust in their leaders and organisations.

Attempts to somehow merge the exit and voice positions, through the market socialist model, or through the public choice bringing of market 'discipline' to public services, have led to the notion of the quasi-market (LeGrand, 1990), and the review of quasi-markets, such as the revamped community care structure, in terms of mixes of exit and voice (Taylor et al, 1992).

What such a model does not do is to explain why so many people appear not to be able or willing to take advantage of these avenues for protest. In reality, people may not benefit from the availability of exit from markets because they may not even be there because of cash, or rely on what they have, and so cannot exit without dire consequences. In many cases, users of social and health services are exactly in this position. It is not easy to either perceive of great involvement in forms of voice such as complaint or such limited forms of consultation as are available to the public.

The exit, voice and loyalty model of alternatives in individual action appear to be based on pluralist assumptions, that there is always some way forward for everyone in liberal democratic society, and nobody can possibly be left out. Such a position ignores the very poor power positions many citizens and consumers are actually in. If there is concern about democracy, efficient allocation or equality, then an important measure is the extent to which people are or feel, denied the possible ways forward, whether it be exit, voice, loyalty or another way. These strategies can be conceived of as 'powers for' but could easily become 'powers against' if they are difficult to use and lack of use is interpreted as lack of interest, rather than low perceived power position, or lack of belief in the power of the strategy.

Lyons and Lowery (1986) have usefully further extended the exit/voice dichotomy to include neglect, which they see as "withdrawal into alienation, cynicism and distrust". With only a minority of voters voting in local elections, and arguably few people complaining where there is a grievance, the whole issue of why people do and do not participate is as important as the different mechanisms for participation and protest enabled by major economic and political strategies. Of course this question is circular, because the same political strategies will have major implications for the willingness of people to participate. Exit and voice can be seen as two strategies for objection and attempting to promote change, while what is missing from the analysis is what people go through in deciding to use either or not bothering at all.

Psychology and identity

The exit/voice model has been taken on board by Tajfel (1981) as analogous to aspects of social identity theory in social psychology. This theory has been developed to look at racism, ethnocentrism and stereotypes, but is used here to look at participation generally. Tajfel saw interindividual and intergroup behaviour as being different ends to a continuum, as far as interpersonal behaviour was concerned. He sees people identifying with groups as part of their own identity and theorises reasons for that identification and the extent of it. He suggests a continuum between the individual idea of social mobility and the group idea of social action, as responses to problems.

Tajfel saw individual notions of identity as coming from a personal and a social process. He concentrates on the social side, basic to which were individuals working out the groups they were members of. Tajfel saw a process of individual social mobility happening where individuals, from their own and others' perceptions of attributions of groups, decided they would and could respond to dissatisfaction with existing group membership by moving to another group that was perceived as more highly valued. By 'group' could be meant wide categories, such as class and race. For many people entry to a higher valued group was not viable, but individuals could decide to join with others to improve the value of their existing group and to take joint action to improve their lot or at least to make more positive the perception of group membership. Such social action may be more viable for most people. Tajfel saw 'social comparisons', a basic psychological mechanism of comparing values of groups, as essential to such a process.

Tajfel analysed stereotypes in terms of 'ingroups' and 'outgroups', as seen from membership of the 'ingroup'. As people's social identity came from group membership, he saw the nearer one came to the intergroup, rather than the interindividual extreme of his continuum, the more extensive the rivalry and belief in superiority of one's own group, along some dimension. The interindividual extreme is direct person to person contact. In the intergroup extreme individuals never come in contact with each other, and members of opposite groups only know each other as undifferentiated members of other groups. Hence the lack of individual contact, and reinforcement of group membership based on race in apartheid in South Africa, reinforced racism and intercommunal violence.

The nearer a social situation is to the intergroup extreme, the stronger tendency there will be for members of the ingroup to treat members of the outgroup as undifferentiated and to make stereotypic attributions to individual members in terms of value judgements and emotional significance, and the more uniformity of behaviour of ingroup members toward the outgroup. As an extreme of intergroup behaviour, bombing undifferentiated members of an outgroup can be seen in stark intergroup terms and can reinforce the ingroup identity as in war, and not cause the personal problems of interindividual assault.

Basic to group membership is the belief that membership of the group makes a positive contribution to the individual's self image. The number and variety of social situations that the individual sees as relevant to his/her group membership is seen as being a function of the clarity of awareness that they are a member of a group (cognitive factor), the extent of positive or negative evaluations associated with membership (evaluative), and extent of emotional investment (emotional factor).

The theory of social comparisons suggests that people continually compare the value of their group with other groups. Tajfel suggested two group solutions to problems of low individual estimation of existing group value: to change beliefs and interpretation of attributes of one's own group to justify or make acceptable initially unwelcome features, or to engage in social action to lead to desirable changes in the situation.

Tajfel put such group solutions at the 'voice' end of his spectrum, while individual mobility to other groups was placed at the 'exit' end. Both exit and voice were available in certain situations – limited social mobility and active group membership at the same time, reflecting that we may be members of several groups, which provides social identity and different forms of protest at wider social situations.

While Tajfel does not discuss 'neglect', he does raise the possibility of people not being actively involved in either social mobility or social action. The tenor of his view appears to be that people will opt for the simpler option and stay in existing groups and hope for change. But Tajfel also suggests that 'outgroups' are important to the identity of the 'ingroup'. The growing 'underclass' can be seen as being rejected by other groups. People may not actively choose to be members, but Tajfel's theory does allow for them to develop a sense of pride, as a group on their own terms, that can be quite negative, but perhaps important, as far as the dominant norms of society as a whole are concerned.

Users and carers in community care may similarly have the role of 'outgroup', and as such, are important to the survival of the existing 'ingroup' of professionals and managers. Members of such an outgroup may be invited to meet the ingroup for consultation, but there may be a lack of belief in, and perhaps hostility to, their membership. The new group may hold a hope for change through the interindividual relations that Tajfel saw as essential in overcoming intergroup conflict. Because of a lack of credibility, measured by the emotional, cognitive and evaluative factors mentioned earlier, such a group may not be able to keep its membership. A 'social comparison' may question the value of such a group compared to other means of change, or no change. The suggestion is that there has to be an emotional and sincere commitment to carers' and users' presence in participation and that it should be a positive and meaningful experience for them, not just the presence of a forum.

Tajfel can be criticised for presenting a theory that effectively rationalises existing power structures, that he sees the reason for their existence as a result of individual actions rather than political and economic forces. An alternative position is that in his analysis he presents possibilities for change by identifying different group and individual approaches that can defy traditional power relations.

A deeper problem with Tajfel may be his optimism, that people will find some way of digging themselves out of situations, through a group or individual approach. He does not address either those who are or feel unable to take exit or voice roads, or where people choose an active approach in response to a negative situation, and this does not work.

A reality with community care is that new policies do not automatically renew people. There may be years of failure of public service support, and years of the feeling of stigma in needing to approach public services. If there is no real material change will we see further bewilderment, cynicism, alienation and neglect? The current rhetoric may be for change but reality may continue to disappoint. Moreover, contrary to Tajfel, at present, it is not easy to see many people with learning disabilities or their carers taking either the individual social mobility or the group change path.

There may not be a simple answer. Tajfel suggests that much of his individual–group dichotomy is based on peoples' attributions and beliefs rather than necessarily reality, so attempts to boost the perceived value of groups themselves leads to some resolution. He also suggests that the closer a process gets to the individual level, the less will group stereotypes (such as, perhaps, the view of social services as stigmatic) be asserted.

The current community care reforms threaten to change such resources as Community Learning Disability Teams (CLDTs): a flexible, relatively easy access and increasingly valued service in many areas. With such teams there is evidence that individual contact and a preventative approach has broken down the stigma of usng social services and health provision, through both a more personal level of negotiating access to resources and more group/community development oriented policies. Brown and Wistow (1990), however, suggest that even with community teams, only a minority of people with learning disabilities receive a personal service. In areas where a higher level of community development is seen as central to the work of CLDTs, more are seen as benefiting. The group identity encouraged by such an approach may provide a more positive approach to change than the individual identity approach of the personal service. Nevertheless, for many, developing new policies (whether it be CLDTs or market-based reforms) may have merely reinforced a view of little change. There may be a better chance of a service, but perhaps, and particularly with the market reforms, at the price of having to be a member of possibly a low value group, those who have to be more rigorously assessed by a stigmatising social services department.

Tajfel might see answers to this in two forms:

- you individually achieve membership of a different group (possibly those who can afford to purchase their own care);

- or, you join with others in the same position to force a less stigmatising service or make political changes to the structure of welfare provision.

There are major problems with carers and users doing either. A corollary of the position of disabled people in society is their poverty, and that affects carers too, so the first option is not readily available. The second option is also problematic. While there are growing numbers of carers and users involved in social movements, there are still major problems in advocacy, self-advocacy and mobility that are crucial to voice, quite apart from the low value that many carers may see to being a member of a group that is still lowly valued in society.

So what questions may come out of social identity theory that will be relevant to this study? Social action is one way forward. Willingness to join in consultation patterns, or to accept the role given to them by government may depend on the willingness of people to be seen as members of such all encompassing groups as 'users and carers'. Or are forms of group action that may lead to more wholesale changes and a more positive group identity preferred to the government's agenda? Equally important will be the perception of individual mobility. How permeable are boundaries of other groups that may not be valued so lowly? If we accept Tajfel's individual mobility – group social action continuum – then the questions about empowerment may be:

- Do you accept the role for disabled people and their carers identified by government and social services?

- What alternatives may there be?

- Can these be achieved by getting together as a group or are they in your individual hands?

- Do consultation procedures consider your voice and your group's voice to have the same importance as other members?

In terms of this study any movement toward group or individual approaches may be a measure of how far participants have come in improving their own power position.

Psychology and power

There is a 'health warning' to be had in considering psychological theories. There is an argument within psychology that 'naive experimentalism' has become predominant, with an overview of people as automatons or mere information processors, rather than active beings. Harré (1993) proposed moving social psychology from an old perspective of seeing people merely as stimuli to one of active and knowledgeable participants. Such a perspective is alive elsewhere in psychology, with a move to incorporate an understanding of cognitive processes (particularly how we make various sorts of attributions in perceiving the world) onto formerly mechanical or computer analogies, or positions based on sometimes controversial studies of animal behaviour. There is also a long standing debate between the psychodynamic position and experimentalists. The former are often accused of highly theoretical analyses of unobservable phenomena based on minimal data, but such representations could be shown to be at least an attempt to define psychological issues on a very personal and feeling level, issues that experimentalists had not, until recently, taken seriously.

Such debates are relevant elsewhere in the social sciences. Theory around policy has also tended to be posed at an impersonal level. This has recently been challenged – particularly by feminists. Studies looking at the very personal position of women carers in community care policy have shown how they, in effect, carry the burden of public policy in this area (Ungerson, 1987; Dalley, 1988).

Part of that debate may be the use ·of psychology itself. Psychodynamic theory has been a major basis to social work, with the work of Bowlby often seen as emphasising the child-rearing role of women in the family, although contemporary developmental psychologists, such as Schaffer, raised an alternative position of the importance of multiple care-takers. The issue may not be so much the role of psychological theory in oppression, as under what circumstances particular theories become predominant, and this may be a question of ideology and power.

There are new alternatives developing in psychology theory. For instance, feminist psychologists (eg, Kitzinger, 1991) have used

Foucault's analysis of power as historical, universal and limiting to develop their own perspectives of psychology in a way that promotes their own differences and interests.

Melanie Klein

While theories derived from experimental psychology are used in this study, there are theories derived from other areas of psychology that may be equally valid. Smith and Brown (1992) looked at normalisation principles from a psychodynamic point of view, using Melanie Klein's notions of the importance of infancy, and how we are thrown back into an infantile internal world at the time of stress. Caring is seen as re-creating conflicts between the carer and the cared-for that started in early childhood when the child was dominated by two feelings: the libidinal (life giving) and the aggressive (death dealing).

> She swings between feeling that she can control other people, notably her mother as the source of food, and feeling powerless and hopeless as her needs are acknowledged or unmet. At the earliest stage the infant cannot distinguish clearly between herself and others and builds up an inner world peopled by her own impulses (good and bad) and the significant people (objects) in her life. Because of the perceived power of the aggressive instinct, the infant's inner world may be felt to be a battlefield, containing many people whom she has damaged and who have damaged her.

Smith and Brown see institutions as the repository of such conflicts, with disabled people becoming the focus of projected images within society. Community care releases these difficult feelings from the institution, and provides new policy and practice issues that have not been faced up to in the safety of the institution. Smith and Brown see the interest in user participation as being part of this picture.

Powerlessness and power, in this view, have both been essential feelings since infancy, but this conflict between life and death continues throughout life: powerlessness balanced by feelings of control. A criticism of this approach is that it over-individualises power. The wider picture of the existence of political, economic and social power is ignored. But Melanie Klein's picture does describe and analyse the emotions around care and of power in a way that experimental and behavioural psychological approaches do not. A larger problem is how we can observe the theorised processes so that they can be used in an experimental study. This issue is avoided here by taking an alternative route in attempting to find theories that bring the behavioural and the cognitive together.

Helplessness

As a theory that originally came from behavioural experiments on humans and animals, including electric shocks on dogs, Seligman's (1975) 'learned helplessness' theory comes from a range of psychological theories that have tended to be rejected by many for humane reasons.

While Tajfel's social psychology theory may tell us something about the processes that are available for change, by the individual, and through individual membership of a group, it does not tell us very much about the processes behind Lyons and Lowery's 'neglect', the withdrawal into alienation and cynicism, that may be key to understanding empowerment. Seligman's theory of helplessness as a learned basis to depression and wider social problems has been used in mental health circles as a description of the environmental difficulties faced by people with mental health problems and as a theory of causation of depression. It has also been taken by the political right as supporting evidence in seeing the welfare state as a disempowering, dependency-producing policy. Seligman himself has rejected such an interpretation, while seeing the need for people who suffer from powerlessness and helplessness to be supported in empowering themselves as a way out of conditioned helplessness. A further criticism (Rees, 1991) of helplessness theory is that it can be seen as blaming the victim, and seeing the problem in terms of individual dysfunction rather than social processes, although behaviourists tend to see individual behaviour as caused by environmental events.

Seligman's theory of learned helplessness stems from controversial experiments with dogs. In a laboratory dogs were given electric shocks no matter what action they took to avoid them, and they eventually gave up doing anything. They were seen as suffering from 'learned helplessness'. In early formulations of his theory Seligman (1975) saw direct comparisons with human depressives. Seligman recognised the problems of deducing human action from animal studies in later formulations of his theory (Abramson, Seligman and Teasdale, 1978) that have emphasised human cognitive functioning, in particular, the notions of internal and external attribution and attributional style. These notions refer to 'social attribution' theory within social psychology. Various theoreticians (see, for example, Hewstone and Antaki, 1988) have tried to analyse the interpretations we give to the causes for observable and unobservable phenomena. One such theory sees the possibility of internal and external causation being attributed by different people for the same event, that it is our fault or an outside influence if something goes wrong. This area of research has tried to identify why and under what circumstances we make such internal or external attributions. One variation on this theory (Abramson, Seligman and Teasdale, 1978; Peterson and Seligman, 1984) sees people as forming attributional styles, with a socially learned tendency (ie, based on past experience) to see causation externally or internally, positively or negatively. This may lead to a 'depressive style' of making attributions in response to events, where there have been consistent negative experiences of those events.

The updated theory (Abramson, Seligman and Teasdale, 1978) concerning depression causation includes four elements:

- an uncontrollable event,

- an attributional style (that may be depressive) determining attribution for that particular event,

- prediction of future occurrence of uncontrollable events,

- events in question to represent highly probable negative outcomes and/or very improbable positive outcomes.

Seligman's response is the regaining of control over outcomes. The reformulated theory that emphasises the importance of attributions and attributional style (Abramson, Seligman and Teasdale, 1978) raises a number of tactics that are not restricted to looking at mental health issues. In brief, they suggest the following:

A. Reduce likelihood of negative outcomes, and increase positive outcomes. This may mean improving services and service responses while making contact with helping personnel more of a positive experience.

B. Reduce aversiveness of highly negative outcomes and reduce desirability of highly desired outcomes, eg, assist re-evaluation. There could be both political and educational aspects to this. A problem with reducing desirability of favoured outcomes is that this can be seen as reinforcing class distinctions and existing power relations: making people happier with them rather than real change in oppressive situations. Arguably this has always been an aim in liberal democratic politics.

C. Change expectation from uncontrollability to controllability. This could mean better use of training and community development, but it is in contradiction with the last possible response.

D. Change attributions for failure or success, from internal to external attributions. You are not the problem but the system has minimised your opportunities. This must be changed. It may be a question of political education but to what extent is this in contradiction with response B?

What is the relation of learned helplessness theory to user and carer empowerment? Despite its narrow basis in behavioural theory and positivist and controversial experimentation, it could be argued that this theory does identify, and helps us understand at least some basis to real individual empowerment in a way that more sociological analyses do not. If it is controllability, accurate predictability, and a history of such processes that are important, then we may be able to predict the processes that do not meet such aims as disempowering. Carers and users in many cases may well feel stigmatised by historically unresponsive and uncontrollable services, and become adverse to asking for support – even being prepared to put up with nothing if the likelihood is of some pain (either through rejection or in the attitude of professionals in providing a perceived stigmatised service). In terms of current community care changes there must be concerns that preventative services (such as CLDTs) that may have countered stigma and brought people back into services (partly through a more positive approach to carers and users) may not be seen as priorities in terms of policy. The proposed responses to helplessness suggest a different policy to current community care reforms, of encouraging positive community development and preventative services.

Questions for a study that arise from such an approach may include:

- How often has your participation led to real change?

- Is it just as likely nothing or something will happen when you participate?

- What has the effect of the success or failure of your interventions been on your frequency of your attendance at meetings?

- Who do you perceive as controlling what happens? you?

- Do you feel it is your fault if nothing happens?

Chapter 3

Perceptions of power

This chapter initially begins to interpret how we may use the theoretical positions looked at in Chapter 2 to analyse power, and particularly the individual's perception of power in certain circumstances. The attempt here is to see how useful the theories are for practice. As an example, the circumstances investigated here are services for people with learning disabilities in one Metropolitan Borough, and the individuals: the carers, users, workers and managers involved in those services. There is then a description of the research methods used here to consider the views of these stakeholders and a report on the research findings.

A brief background

Since 1983, the Borough's services for people with learning disabilities have been coordinated on a joint health/social services basis – through joint planning teams at policy level, and through community teams at front-line level. These are staffed by a social worker, community nurse and support workers at each of five localities in the borough. These are supported by a consultant psychiatrist and a team of psychologists, both based centrally, and by other social services workers providing specific services. There is also a small hospital unit, built in the late seventies.

At the time of this study the focus of these teams was changing from one of open access community support to a more focused assessment in line with the demands of the NHS and Community Care Act 1990, and social services' decision to organise its personnel along purchaser/provider lines.

Power and learning disability services

There have been a number of analyses of the relative power of individuals in such services. Tyne (1982) saw the medical profession dominating these services and any change continuing to reflect such power positions. Barnes (1991) saw professionals generally as disempowering disabled people. It was suggested in Chapter 1 that the new community care arrangements following the NHS and Community Care Act 1990 gave more power to managers, through greater emphasis on budget control. The Audit Commision (1992a, b) saw the basis of the legislation as an attempt to move power from service providers to users.

Normalisation (eg, Wolfensberger, 1980) has been a major philosophy in the development of learning disability services, an attempt to change the way people with learning disabilities are seen and a philosophy behind the move away from institutions. This has been seen by Dalley (1992) as forcing people with learning disabilities into narrow patterns of conformity divorced from their individuality. Normalisation and concepts of what is normal were seen by Foucault (1979a) as ways power is operated, so historically we are all formed into narrow definitions of acceptability.

Observing power

There is little shared analysis of power in learning disability services but this has not prevented policy decisions being made as if there was a shared analysis. This study is about how individuals themselves perceive their power position, their use of power, and how they perceive power affecting them. There are likely to be major problems in attempting to look at power issues from any notion of neutrality, and this may help explain why there is no shared analysis. It can be argued from a number of the theoretical perspectives of power, already outlined, that we all have a power position and we take this wherever we go, although we may draw different power positions from different aspects of our individual identity and membership of different social groups (Tajfel, 1981). It is suggested that whether it is known or not known to people we speak to, we still carry such a power position with us. Academic researchers may be seen by the interviewee as carrying the power of publicity, prestige, possibly hidden bonuses if there is cooperation and possibly hidden debits of reporting back to a more powerful person. In researchers' own minds there may be the power of who is funding the research and future employment needs. Members of organisations studying their own organisation may possess the power of knowledge and relationships already made with relevant interviewees, and the possible debit of being in a known power position relative to those interviewees. One may hope that the power position, as far as professionals interviewing carers and users are concerned, is seen as 'power for' rather than 'power over' but that has to be a subjective interpretation and is certainly not guaranteed.

A further issue may be that talking to people about power issues may actually be educational and may begin to change how individuals perceive and respond to power.

Rees (1991) actively advocates the use of 'biography' to enable individuals, particularly users of social services, to understand and confront power issues through an analysis of how their life histories have been influenced by their power positions in different circumstances.   Marxist theory includes the notion of 'false consciousness' in which the 'working class' are seen, through ideology reflecting the relations of production, as being fooled into working against their own interests in continuing to support those relations. Marxists see the power situation changing through workers understanding their real power position.

So, in looking at power, neutrality may not be possible, and we may merely be observing a snapshot of a view of power at one particular moment, in a changing scene, that the interviewers themselves are helping to change.

Interviews

A basic issue is the extent to which perceptions of power positions are shared, and how power is perceived personally. Accordingly, the author has chosen a comparative and qualitative methodology. While a quantitative study may give us statistically significant data on differences between participants in their views of power, there have to be some agreed notions from which to ask the right questions. We are not presently at that stage. Rather, we still have to find out what questions are of concern to participants, and are important in looking at individual perceptions of power, and empowerment. Moreover, the 'raison d'être' of this study itself is that power has individual meaning, and this study attempts to seek such meanings out with a view to forging clearer models and methods of empowerment.

The author interviewed two senior managers and three workers representing health and social services involvement, and five carers and three service users, all in one metropolitan borough. The questions that arose from the discussion of different theories in Chapter 2 were refined and used as a semi-structured interview schedule. These schedules were designed to highlight the three areas discussed previously:

- direct and indirect power (based on Lukes [1974] and Foucault [1979a])

- strategies, based on exit and voice (Lyons and Lowery [1986])

- psychological approaches (Seligman [1975] and Tajfel [1981])

The emphasis is, rather than seeing these three areas as separate, to see them as enabling a study of power from different perspectives. Obviously the small sample particularly of carers and users interviewed means that we need to be careful not to over-generalise in our descriptions of findings. However, a focus of this study is to demonstrate how me may use our theoretical structure and to use this to make some comparison between stakeholders' viewpoints.

Findings

The aim of this study is to seek individual perceptions of power. The interview schedules used are reprinted in the appendix (see pp 75-77). These were designed around the theoretical perspectives identified in Chapter 2.

Two questions arise:

- are these theories descriptive of how power works?

- have they been useful in helping us understand more about how individuals perceive power?

First of all, the author is going to take a general look at the views of power that have come from the interviews and will then analyse the data in terms of the three-fold analysis presented in Chapter 2.

Perceptions of power

From the findings:

- there are contradictions and tensions in the exercise of power

- there is little evidence of a shared view of empowerment – rather, this was interpreted very personally by participants, in terms of their individual power.

- *There are tensions in one person's empowerment being another person's disempowerment.* Carers were seen by other carers and workers as empowering themselves by individual assertiveness and group campaigning. One carer and one community nurse saw carer involvement in both local Quality Action Groups (QAGs) and in the political arena as important to empowering carers. The potential effect of this on their guardianship of users was seen by other workers as, in practice, disempowering, because this was used to deny independence to the user. A health psychologist commented that collusion between carers and workers prevented decisions being made by users. The social services social worker commented how the better organised carers in the wealthier part of the borough effectively preempted resources from carers and users in poorer areas.

- *Certain actions are seen as empowering by one actor, but disempowering by others because of different understandings of empowerment.* An example of this was the belief by a health authority manager that he was empowering users by moving them to the private sector. This was seen by front-line workers as disempowering, as in reality it was forced for administrative reasons on users who were perceived as having little choice in where they went.

- *There were also differences between empowering theory and disempowering practice.* Managers and other players saw the development of user and carer participation as empowering, but all players also saw the actual process of participation as disempowering through incomprehensible agendas and unwelcoming membership. These were perceived as so difficult that even one carer, whose job had been organising such meetings, reported difficulty in participation. Similarly, the development by managers of QAGs are seen as empowering in principle by carers and workers, but not in their actual operation, where the failure of managers to attend or to respond to participants' concerns was seen by carers as disempowering. Another carer cast doubts on whether the committees of consultation she was a member of were part of the decision-making process. Rather, she felt they actually prevented decisions being made, and they were organised in ways that prevented relevant issues being discussed.

- *There were tensions between different roles of the same person.* The local presence of front-line workers was seen by carers and workers as empowering them, but they were seen in other ways as disempowering. A worker thanked health managers for empowering him by basing him in a locality. Carers saw the worker as part of a decentralised bureaucracy and as accepting bureaucratic limits. Workers felt that they empowered users and carers through advocacy and through assertiveness training, but users reported frustration. One user saw workers "only supporting him when it suited workers". One carer spoke of workers empowering when they gave advice against the interest of their employers, but the health psychologist felt that they were more likely to collude with managers or carers against the interest of users, for instance, when workers left users in a residential home they wanted to move from.

- *Users appeared to have least control of all stakeholders.* Their actions to empower themselves could have the opposite effect. One user spoke of needing to speak up to get what he wanted, but historically this had sometimes been taken negatively, for example, by residential workers who had punished him for this. Users appeared to have to go to greater lengths to become empowered, and to depend more on the power of others. A worker suggested that the most immediate response to users' needs had been after someone had been scalded in the bath. Workers saw themselves as empowering where they could offer users a choice in living arrangements, but the users that the author spoke to denied being offered real choices in such important situations.

- *There was little evidence of a shared view of what empowerment is, or of a shared value of the importance of empowerment.* To the health authority manager, empowerment was about deinstitution-alisation and his freedom, for example, to manage complaints and resources. The community nurse saw empowerment about his own freedom from the disempowerment of the hospital bureaucracy. Workers said that they wanted independence and availability of choice for users, but admitted that practice was more restrictive, and perhaps more geared to the views of parents or their managers. Workers seemed to see empowerment in terms of their own assertiveness and their ability to protect, or to restrict the independence of, users. Users wanted a different set of 'powers' – support when they needed it; for their wishes to be taken seriously, ie, when they wanted to move; and access to information and facilities kept from them by petty rules made by managers and workers. Empowerment as a concept appeared to be interpreted very personally by all stakeholders rather than as a policy requirement, even when that interpretation could deny empowerment to another party.

The above examples give a flavour of some of the paradoxes and tensions in perceptions of empowerment. Figures 1 and 2 (see pp 38-41) summarise those points and take them further, reflecting the following discussion, which uses the three-fold analysis from Chapter 2.

Figure 1: Summary of views on how stakeholders empower and disempower

Stakeholder	Empowers by	Disempowers by
Managers	■ Closing and moving people out of institutions. ■ Setting up user-friendly consultation. ■ Influencing politicians. ■ Developing resources. ■ Support to front-line workers. ■ Negotiating complaints. ■ Implementing market systems can help individuals through enabling strategies. ■ Policy decisions on joint work in CLDTs between health/social services departments. ■ Accepting the official way may not be the best.	■ Moving people for administrative reasons/with limited consultation. ■ Top-down implementation of policy. ■ Ignorance of front-line activity. ■ Specifying ways things are to be done, including using own language and controlling agendas. ■ Denial of substantive rights or methods for front-line workers to obtain resources (eg, identifying needs). ■ Not participating in QAGs, etc. ■ Not valuing role of carers in decisions. ■ Limiting resources.
Front-line workers	■ Local presence. ■ Direct contact with carers. ■ Advice given to carers and users in QAGs, etc. ■ Ability to advocate for users where to take risk of giving advice against interest of organisation. ■ Enable genuine choice. ■ Advocacy/ assertion training.	■ Decisions being made for users. ■ Deciding own workload. ■ Part of centralised bureaucracy. ■ Fear of own job loss. ■ Only able to offer restricted resources. ■ Accepting bureaucratic limits. ■ Inability to proffer rights. ■ Tendency to collusion with carers and/or managers. ■ Not developing advocacy.

| Carers | ■ Individual assertion.
■ Participation in QAGs, etc.
■ Guardians of users.
■ Pushing own views counters bureaucratic tendency to see carers of low value.
■ Developing group campaigns.
■ Influencing politicians. | ■ Own needs rather than users.
■ Collusion with workers where accept constraints of bureaucracy.
■ Non-participation.
■ Not influencing politicians. |
| Users | ■ Individual assertion (+ve response).
■ Challenging behaviour (+ve response).
■ Membership of advisory groups. | ■ Individual assertion (-ve response).
■ Challenging behaviour (-ve response).
■ Non-participation in groups. |

Figure 2: Summary of views on how stakeholders are empowered
          and disempowered

Stakeholder	Empowered by	Disempowered by
Managers	■ Positive strategies/policies. ■ Choices of approach through market systems. ■ Ability to negotiate complaints. ■ Ability to take strategic decisions. ■ Ability to manage meetings, etc. ■ Budget management means limit on demands.	■ Government policy dictating alternatives. ■ Scruples over helping individuals. ■ Performance monitoring. ■ Committees only operating in particular ways. ■ Lack of local strategy. ■ Power lying elsewhere, eg, health, social security. ■ Carers' power over users.
Front-line workers	■ Localisation policy supporting joint working. ■ Links with carers. ■ Agreement with managers. ■ Independence from medical and administrative interference where rights of carers and users clear. ■ Knowledge of law/procedures used to help. ■ Carers taking up issues raised by workers, which workers have difficulty with. ■ Respect for users.	■ Carers' power over users. ■ Managers making decisions over head and without consulting. ■ Fear of job loss if oppose managers/policy. ■ Being told by managers not to, eg, identify needs. ■ Carer/manager collusion. ■ No response from managers. ■ Ignorance of managers.

Carers	■ Self-assertion. ■ Participation in QAGs, etc. ■ Being guardians of users. ■ Group campaigning. ■ Recognition of positive self-value. ■ Victories in campaigning.	■ Committee procedures. ■ Workers offering no choice. ■ Managers not participating/consultation as paper exercise. ■ Perception of not being valued as partners in decisions. ■ Lack of real rights. ■ Minor players, eg, drivers. ■ Lack of managerial direction. ■ Fear of managerial retribution. ■ Historical professional dominance.
Users	■ Self-assertion. ■ Challenging behaviour. ■ Advocacy training. ■ Enabling workers. ■ Some group meetings.	■ Carers given priority. ■ Workers not listening or giving no choice. ■ User groups as official activity, not users' themselves. ■ Petty rules in residential and day support, prevent access.

Dimensions of power

Lukes' first dimension was about direct power. All four sets of stakeholders tended to suggest that they were not able to have a substantial direct influence, but descriptions of events suggested very direct influences on behaviour and activities by all stakeholders, although the extent of that power varies, as described in the above discussion and in Figures 1 and 2.

Direct power is shown in a number of ways. Carers and users talked of workers making decisions affecting users' lives. One user talked of being moved from one residential home to another with little say in decisions about where he wanted to live. He wanted to stay at home but his parents would not let him. He was given no alternatives to consider, and he felt that social workers and community nurses only helped when it suited them and not when it suited him – they had stopped him getting what he wanted.

Another user also lives in a family household. About 12 months before he had been moved from a small private residential unit, following a history of residential care. This user wanted to leave the previous Home but had had to approach a social worker several times, and angrily, before his request was taken seriously. There had been objections from the proprietor and manager of the Home to the user leaving, and his parents had also tried to stop him, although they lived 30 miles away.

One carer said that a worker had only given him one choice of a day centre. Workers spoke of the power of managers. One social worker pointed to a recent social services managerial decision instructing him not to identify definitive needs, because identifying needs may mean rights to resources. He felt that this instruction disempowered him and users, as the use of legislation and knowledge of welfare rights, etc, were keys to his ability to empower others.

Managers had made policy decisions that had led to a large number of residents moving from the NHS unit to the private sector, while government policy decisions were reported by managers as having directly led to such actions. One health authority manager was concerned at the extent of power that carers had to stop users being resettled, but not about the power of the health authority to resettle, which he clearly saw as a 'power for'.

A CLDT community nurse also felt that he and users were disempowered by managers and carers. He felt that carers had tremendous power over users, and when he tried to act for users independently of carers there were considerable objections from carers.

Positive uses of power

There was also evidence of such direct power being used positively, whereas Lukes' tenor is to see power negatively. The community nurse felt that he had also been personally empowered by carers and managers. The strategy of localisation and joint working had freed him from the managerial constraints of the hospital hierarchy.

Carers and workers reported the support given by workers to carers in the development of their assertiveness. One carer described how a residential respite care resource had been the result of an assertive approach by carers. One carer felt that her belief in assertiveness came from an awareness that carers had historically been more influential than was realised by carers. Pressure in the past had successfully led to the development of resources, including special schools and centres. Most recently this particular carer had used her local knowledge, including information from front-line workers, to campaign for a residential respite care resource. This included incisively questioning health managers at a public meeting in a way that undermined their argument not to provide such a resource. Subsequently, such a resource was made available. This carer felt that her power had come from superior knowledge about needs and locality, which carers did have. She felt that challenging managerial power was a key to obtaining resources. She and other carers had to insist on being represented on a recent day care review after being told that this was only a "professional matter". This carer saw front-line workers' lack of power also coming from such an attitude and their unwillingness to challenge it because of fear. As a carer she had no job to lose and so challenged managers. She recognised that few carers had the knowledge to use the system to their benefit.

One user felt that he had got what he wanted (a move to a new home) by pushing for this. All stakeholders appeared to have the ability to make a positive use of such power as they had.

The non-use of positive power

Within both positive and negative examples there is evidence of power being directly used in some way by all stakeholders, as shown in Figure 1, whereas Lukes seems to suggest power coming from a single dominant source. However, the four groups of stakeholders may not hold power equally, with managers and carers seemingly able to exert rather more influence over the lives of users than workers and users themselves. It is not clear whether they actually have more power, or whether they use their power to different extents, or alternatively more easily recognise the power they have. There was criticism from all stakeholders toward the other stakeholders as to their use of positive power, while each had their own reason as to why they did not use power positively.

All workers saw themselves as only able to influence outcomes if their views coincided with those of managers. They also felt their ability to enable users was severely limited by carers.

The carers of an 18-year-old woman with a severe learning disability felt that front-line workers had little influence. Managers did have influence but rarely used it – rather, there was considerable 'buck passing'. They felt that the real basis to power was money and a lack of it prevented their daughter's needs being met.

These carers thought that recent health managerial changes had reduced the ability of health professionals to make decisions. In the past, there were particular clinicians, consultants in particular, who would make decisions. This had become more diffuse, and it was difficult to know who could be approached to make a decision.

One user was very critical of workers' ability to help, as quoted earlier, seeing this as only when it was in the worker's interests. One manager was critical of carers for preventing the resettlement process, while two workers were critical of managers for their dominance over such a process. The general perception appeared to be that the dominant use of direct power came from carers and managers, rather than from workers and users.

Lukes' second dimension suggested that negative power was used more indirectly with processes reflecting traditional power relations, through 'a mobilisation of bias'. In this study, committees were reported by at least one member of each of the four groups of stakeholders as operating in a language of their own. Agendas and procedures did not allow different issues to be raised or existing issues to be understood by users and carers. This was the case not just for those unused to committees but for those who had considerable experience elsewhere. The price of entry was high, with a health authority manager who perceived carers and users as having to be more representative than professionals. The social services manager saw such committees as 'patronising' carers and users, but also saw access to management as 'needing to be managed' to reduce the demand on their time and workers' time.

Carers spoke of having to persevere to get their messages across, but also reported managers not turning up to QAGs, for example, as they became successful in their assertiveness. There was a belief by one carer in a councillor–manager axis that prevented other voices being heard. Her experience was of councillors taking the manager's side rather than the more independent stance that she had expected. This seems to represent a 'mobilisation of bias' by managers and policy makers. One user spoke of workers helping him when it was in their interests but not when he wanted help, and carers described the limited choice offered by workers. This suggests that front-line workers also wielded indirect power through having their own agenda, displayed through selectively offering choice or responding to requests by users. This agenda was not easily accessible to users who had to challenge in some way to be heard, and this was sometimes perceived as aggressive behaviour by workers and carers. A 'mobilisation of bias' can also be seen in the collusion, reported by one worker, between carers and workers that prevented users' needs being prioritised.

There appear to be many examples of Lukes' second dimension of 'a mobilisation of bias', not in terms of a single power source but of different power gradients, for example, workers ignoring users' requests and managers running meetings in such a way as to prevent carers' and users' involvement. With indirect power there were also positives, with workers using QAGs, etc, to give advice at odds with the interests of their employers, and QAGs often beginning to speak a different language from managers. There was also a view, however, that this was still incomprehensible to users, who were a victim of indirect power here too. If an analysis of direct power showed workers had little power, then indirect power here may show how workers do influence, but continue to leave users disempowered.

Lukes' third power dimension was more ideological in nature and concerned the possibility of people acting against their own objective interests. This is more difficult to identify, and to distinguish from Foucault's 'fourth power dimension', of power being historically formed and reinforced structurally rather than by specific groups and individuals. One user did talk about staying in a care situation he was unhappy with, but he stayed because he had no support in moving, and this is an example of someone being forced to act against their interests.

There was evidence of rights being avoided, and this appears to be because of an unstated negative attitude to such rights, from an underlying ideology. All users appeared sceptical and/or ignorant of complaints procedures. This may reflect the lack of information given to users that managers and workers do have the ability to give, but also a general negative aura around either managers giving such information or users making use of it. One health authority manager expressed pride in dealing with complaints before they were made official, and hence stopping them being made, as if it was 'not done' for complaints to be made at all. Similarly, the lack of knowledge of rights and the imposition of petty rules, such as over the use of telephones, access to files and bedtimes in residential care, reported by users at a self-advocacy day, shows ideology and its impact in terms of direct, if arbitrary, power.

One user was concerned "not to break the law", so everything had to be officially done, for example, in meetings, and he had to keep quiet at times, he felt, as his wish to move may have been "against the law". This user seemed to feel that social workers were policeman who had the possibility of helping him but also of locking him up. He said that he had experienced both while in residential care and had relied on his personal relationship with workers to stop him being locked up. It took him a while to realise whether he was "breaking the law" or not. He felt his own ability to ask questions and to assert his views had helped him get what he wanted, but this had been taken negatively by some workers.

This may reflect ideological expectations about his behaviour as a 'handicapped person'. Such an ideological framework, based on traditional power relations, may also be reflected in the fear that all workers reported they had for their job if they spoke out, and the fear of retribution, reported by one carer, if carers complained. The social services worker reported that the bottom line, as far as he was concerned, was his ability to pay his mortgage, which could be affected if he said the wrong thing at the wrong time. One carer saw her power coming from her freedom from such constraints. She spoke of the continual professional power, from the birth of a disabled child, over carers and people with disabilities, which was difficult to challenge.

Foucault's notion of 'disciplinary power' appears to be reflected by the degree of fear and difficulties in challenging the status quo that appears to run throughout these services for people with learning disabilities.

To summarise, direct power (Lukes' first face) was seen as being strongest for carers and managers, and indirect power (Lukes' second face) for workers and managers. Users were put into positions where they acted against their interests (Lukes' third face), while ideological influences cast a climate of fear over the ability of all stakeholders to challenge the status quo even when their procedural rights to do so were clear (Foucault).

Exit and voice

This section discusses strategies that may exist for complaint and choice. Exit is seen as the market's ability to offer choice, in terms of offering an alternative product if the customer is dissatisfied. In this study managers were enthusiastic about the choice market systems would bring, but other stakeholders were rather sceptical. As there was no substantial experience of the new systems at the time of interviewing it is difficult to be directly analytical of the process. There were previous experiences where carers and users had attempted to exercise choice. Carers seemed to feel considerable frustration at the lack of responsiveness from the official ways of doing things, and to feel even the procedural rights of complaint and involvement in planning were more apparent than real.

One couple, who are carers, reported frustrations historically at the lack of choice for day services available to their son. Two of the three users had had difficulty in persuading professionals to take seriously either choices that existed, or their rights to exercise that choice, when they wished to move. Users appeared initially perplexed by the author's questions in this area, almost as if there was a fear in answering them.

One user said that he had been given no choice of possibilities at the various times he had moved. Indeed, at each step, he had been denied the choice he actually wanted. He had wanted to move from his present home, but had no cooperation in trying to do so.

Another user said that he had to push social workers and against the wishes of both home owners and his parents to be offered an alternative. He had difficulty knowing where he stood and had to rely on his attempts to develop positive relationships with professionals. He regularly felt that his ability to ask questions was not valued by professionals, but he felt that he had to keep asking to get what he wanted.

Workers were reported by users and carers as only suggesting one choice where they were involved, and denying genuine choice when this was requested, or needed. This was seen as not necessarily happening through direct refusal to offer choices, but through deliberate non-involvement of workers. Managers saw this process as part of the service-led process of social services, which emphasised the use of existing council-owned services. But even when a choice was possible and was identified by carers, this seemed to be denied.

Within the new quasi-market, workers complained of being instructed by managers not to identify need because of the possibility that this would give legal rights to a service. The effect of this was to deny access to the exercise of choice under the community care legislation. A senior social services manager felt that if people took rights to assessment seriously, social services was in trouble, so part of the role of workers was to limit expectations.

In so far as it is possible to make comments about the workings of a new system, while it is possible there may be greater choice, most stakeholders other than managers were sceptical that access to that choice would be improved.

Voice refers to the ability to 'voice' the need for change, for instance, through complaining or political action. A social services manager was concerned that use of procedures for complaints, participation, etc, was already limited to those who knew how to shout. Rights could only be procedural, limited to rights to dignity, etc, and not substantive rights, which would overload social services. She felt that case managers and social workers should have a proper advocatorial role, but in cases of conflict, their local government officer role had to come first. The market was seen as solving the substance of many complaints by providing choice and the possibility of moving from one resource to another. Support was given to platforms for voice such as QAGs, while recognition was made of officials speaking a different language from carers and users and limiting their usefulness through procedures.

The health authority manager felt that too often carers' and users' comments were not taken seriously because they were not believed by professionals to be representative, despite professsionals themselves not having to be representative. The health authority manager spoke of the importance of the public meetings that the health authority had organised. However, he said that there were rarely new questions at such meetings, as they had already been dealt with outside the meetings. Similarly, there had been few official complaints made to him, but many informal complaints, which he dealt with informally.

The health psychologist saw the complaints procedure as reactive and not easily accessible. He felt that implicit in the processes for complaining was a lack of respect for complainants, and when complaints were investigated, the professionals' version of events was given more credence than that of carers' or users'. Sometimes, where complaints were used was a matter of manipulation (by some workers), of carers to get what they wanted. The health psychologist also saw the tendency to compromise in informally dealing with complaints, rather than really sorting problems out.

The community nurse had also had problems obtaining copies of the health complaints procedure. He believed that certain carers had shown the advantage of a more confrontative approach in forcing policy change, involving QAGs, but also publicity, lobbying of councillors, and more active use of public meetings. The community nurse saw that users tended to see professionals as very powerful people. Many did challenge their decisions, but this was often written off as 'challenging behaviour' rather than an attempt at voice.

One couple, who were carers, had found that making an official complaint about transport had led to problems with trade unions and to bad relations with drivers. They felt that it had not been worth the complaint.

The health psychologist felt that there was a fear by carers and workers alike that complaining set officials and managers against them in the long run. The community nurse also spoke of the fear that carers had of losing a service if they complained. The social worker feared for his job if he enabled a complaint.

This study suggests that carers, users and workers have a fear and distrust of using processes of voice such as complaints procedures, which restricts their use. This fear does not necessarily reflect a fear of managers. There are wider concerns, such as, of the consequences of complaining for relationships with other players. Carers and users believe that there are considerable constraints on their issues reaching official agendas through complaints procedures.

There were also criticisms of other platforms for voice. Despite some carers' long experience of meetings, they found reports and procedures were difficult to understand and the attitude of officials was such as to treat their lack of understanding of them as the problem rather than the way information was presented. They also felt that officials were not in favour of widespread knowledge of services and procedures for complaining because of the fear of being overwhelmed. This meant that many parents did not know how to complain, and many of those who did were put off by prevarication.

QAGs had been successful, but as carers found their voice, this had been accompanied by a reduced attendance by managers, and meant that it was difficult to take their views further. It was difficult to get certain professionals to take their views seriously anyway. One consultant had responded to a concern with the response that a certain decision was his to make, and not theirs.

Users were sceptical of official 'self-advocacy' groups as being controlled by centre workers and not leading anywhere, while one worker saw users as effectively excluded from QAGs as carers took over. One manager was critical of a carer group for campaigning against a policy, suggesting initially that members would not be welcome as participants in official meetings. Carers felt that the QAGs could be a basis for improving resources but would need to go further than was expected by managers, including campaigning for resources, and being involved in political lobbying. One worker was critical of this as preempting resources. Other workers encouraged carers to lobby, in order to obtain more resources.

The success of voice seems to depend on how it is used. It can be a 'Catch 22' with procedures being supported by managers where this suits managers, but not if carers and users begin to speak up in the way that they had been encouraged to. There are also concerns that a redistribution of power, which voice allows, only offers influence to those carers prepared and able to participate. Existing power structures continue to act on those unwilling or unable to take part, and on those perceived as lower down the power scale, such as users.

To summarise, there are considerable cross currents that run against the use of both exit and voice as strategies for change. It does seem that how far carers and users can benefit from such strategies depends on individual actions and assertiveness.

Psychological definitions

These, as a very brief and incomplete resumé, led to the questions:

- Seligman's learned helplessness: how far do processes not lead to change, or punish people for participating, and hence discourage participants from further involvement?

- Tajfel's social identity theory: how far do people choose individual or group approaches to change as a way of improving their lot, or neither? The choice of approach or whether to change at all is seen as based on one's perception of value in present and possible future groups. Change can happen by the individual moving to a group perceived as better valued, or by improving the value of an existing group through group action.

Inevitably, some of these issues have already been discussed.

In this section there is an attempt to identify three of Seligman's factors: continual negative consequences of involvement, historical uncontrollability of events, and the consequence of apathy and non-involvement as aspects of 'learned helplessness'.

How welcome is involvement? Managers were clear in that they supported the involvement of carers and users in planning groups, although there was some scepticism toward carers organising themselves, particularly where aims contradicted official policies.

Has this involvement been encouraged through positive results? One health authority manager felt that there had been real change through the consultation procedures and public meetings. This had led to the empowerment of those resettled to the independent sector. He felt it important that managers did listen, because people would not come to meetings if they did not. He recognised that carers and users were not always encouraged, that meetings were often organised on professionals' and managers' terms, and he felt that they should be organised more informally. He also felt that there were demands on carers and users to be representative that were not there for professionals. They had to prove themselves as members of the participation group more than professionals and managers.

The senior social services manager saw many professionals and managers in such groups as "patronising carers and users", but felt that managers and professionals with an advocatorial stance took a different and more enabling role. A problem was the difficulty of managers feeling comfortable in communicating, particularly with users with learning disabilities. She saw the opening of the market and the reduced prescribing of outcomes by workers as meaning that it lead to a more positive approach to participation. She did feel it important that carers should be able to affect change but she did not feel able to say whether they actually had in the recent past. The senior social services manager recognised a "responsibility to respond: it was difficult for us to listen ... why should we have the monopoly of good ideas?"

Users were mixed in their reports on their historical ability to control their lives. All three had made attempts at change but this had been rebuffed by parents and/or workers. All three had at some time been frustrated in attempts to receive help with movement to a new home. Two also reported situations where they had been 'told off' for requesting a move. One reported being confused as to how to change, he was frightened of 'breaking the law', and suggested that a lack of clear control as carers/workers gave inconsistent and sometimes punitive responses to his requests. Users were lukewarm to the value of meetings, and had become selective.

Are attempts at change encouraged? Neither of the three users spoken to had been involved in group campaigns and the author had difficulty in explaining what he meant. This in itself suggested a historical negative view towards even learning about how to change. The author attended a user self-advocacy feedback session during the preparation of this project and found a strong message from participants in residential care that there was a need to be released from constraints that prevented them from being treated as people with human rights. These constraints included, for example, a lack of use of a telephone, being allowed access to files, and being allowed to choose own bedtimes. These demands were objected to by certain of the carers present, as "professionals putting ideas into their minds". It may be that many users still have far to go to be accepted as members of campaigning groups, with rights to change their lives.

In decision-making groups control was denied through higher expectations of users being representative of other users than was the case for professionals. The experience of users was of both inconsistent support for moves to take control of their lives, and frequently of negative reactions to such attempts, as when they have attempted to fulfil their own decision to move to a new home.

A lack of control over the environment was widely felt. Carers and workers reported their lack of control over resources. Carers and users reported little choice offered by workers and managers even where they pushed for alternatives. The health psychologist felt that users were only accepted even on QAGs in a token manner and that their views were widely not even responded to. Carers' and users' descriptions of their difficulty in becoming accepted members of consultation groups also suggests the negative consequences of membership.

Seligman's model suggests that participants continue to make attempts at control until the historical experience of lack of control and negative consequences lead them to believe that they cannot control their environment. This is shown by non-participation and apathy. All stakeholders here reported continued active involvement in at least one form of participation. The very small sample interviewed here may be more tenacious than most, as few carers and users are involved in QAGs.

Abramson, Seligman and Teasdale (1978) suggest that those with a negative 'attributional style' give up rather earlier. Those with such a style have a tendency to fatalism formed by their continued negative experience of participation. Many carers have decades of experience in dealing with social and health services and may indeed have given up. A small number of carers have persevered with QAGs and report more control over these, but not necessarily more control over policy, as managers are reported to have responded by not coming to QAGs and reducing the control carers thought they had.

As a behavioural model of participation, the model of 'learned helplessness' appears useful. Its strength may be in the understanding of the need for individuals to control their environment and in avoiding negative consequences of such attempts at control. It is also a model that shows how the more powerful can reinforce the powerlessness of others, and whether intended or not this study suggests that this is happening. Managers appear to want to exert strong influence on the exercise of participation. Groups' opposing policies are actively dissuaded. Attempts by users to exert control are prevented by arbitrary rules, a failure to respond to concerns, and a lack of managerial commitment to participation.

If the basis to control and encouragement is substantive rights and access to resources, then this raises questions for policy. Present quasi-market systems, with the emphasis on narrower priorities, may be leading to a situation where carers have less control over resources. Access under the quasi-market becomes limited to those assessed as eligible by social services officials. This access becomes more restricted as the budget becomes more limited. This is difficult to solve without sufficient resources, but it is not helped if users have not been able to participate in decisions about rationing or use of resources.

Helplessness theory suggests the value of a community work model that allows greater access to services through supporting carers and users in pushing for their share of resources. This model both potentially increases the amount of resources, and carers' and users' confidence in their ability to influence events. But this model may actually be becoming less available as the CLDT approach becomes modified by the rationing and individual model of care management within the quasi-market.

Social identity

Tajfel's 'social identity theory' is based around the comparisons people are seen as making between themselves and others, and the idea that people wish to belong to groups they identify with and value. Crudely summarising the consequences of such comparisons, if people wish for change and they believe that they cannot individually join a more valued group, they will try to alter their existing group.

There appears to be much evidence for carers pushing to improve their status, particularly through group campaigns, but also through their tenacity in forcing consultation groups to accept their views as of at least equal value to professionals and managers. According to workers, managers and workers may also have played a part in this, through the strategy of local joint CLDTs, as this has become based on partnership. Through the CLDT, carer campaigning activity is frequently enabled in a way unplanned by managers, with the benefit of advice from workers. This is seen by carers and workers in this study to benefit workers as well as carers, because workers come to recognise the value of carer action in developing resources.

Carers were increasingly recognising the impact of the group approach, and were clear that they felt unwelcome in official bodies. One couple who were carers were not involved in any of the participation fora. They felt that they should have been involved, but had never been invited, or even encouraged. He was a representative of respite carers on a regional group, and commented on how long it had taken to understand how the meetings worked and the language used. Others had dropped out of the meetings but his persistance had helped improve his chances of being taken seriously, as he felt he had not initially been seen as the equal of professionals by participants. He thought that it was realistic for carers to promote change, although this was hard work.

Workers appeared to have found an avenue for themselves as well as carers in group approaches. The community nurse felt that he encouraged a group approach to resources through the advice he gave to QAG members and other carers and he felt that the minority of carers involved had achieved change in a number of areas. This had developed as carers had taken over the lead of QAGs from managers. To some extent he now felt that it was the "carers' fault" if they did not participate. He felt that carers should be forced to attend regular meetings if they wanted resources, as he felt that there had been a loss of battles for resources because of a low level of active support for such resources by carers.

The users had mixed feelings about participation groups. They all felt that they were treated as full members of their house groups, and they all gave examples of things changing after they had said something at those groups.   This was not true of the day centre participation group, which they saw as a waste of time (the two involved had dropped out of these groups as they did not value them).

One carer had a deep belief that the only way to improve the perceived value of carers was through assertiveness and group campaigning, which both improved peoples' image of themselves and was more likely to lead to real change.   The campaigning group itself can help members understand procedures and actively participate, but can also overcome the ubiquitous view: "we are lucky to have what we have got" that reflected inertia by carers and was encouraged by professionals.   Such gratefulness meant that many carers and users had hidden needs, which campaigning groups were more able to put back on the agenda.

This view was shared by another couple who were carers.   Despite one of this couple's professional involvement with the regional health authority, he felt a tendency to be seen as lower in value.   They saw advocacy and assertiveness training as important, but if they, as fairly assertive people, had difficulty with processes, then more was needed.   They felt that the group campaigning approach was key here.

The senior social services manager commented that a group had been campaigning for a new day centre to be built, which managers were against.   She initially suggested that it would be wrong to encourage such a group, because they were actively opposed to a policy decision, but later suggested that they could be engaged in discussion as a reflection of the advocacy and carer involvement such a group meant, which itself was in keeping with policy.   However, it did seem that acceptance of such groups was not automatic or valued but had to be proved.

One problem with Tajfel's theory is a presumption that it is easy to identify change and the choice of a valued route.   The health psychologist thought it difficult to describe what 'real change' would be as there was no shared vision.   There was a tendency for carers to be reactive and defensive toward existing resources and this prevented the development of new facilities that users may perceive as more valued. This left users disempowered.

Tajfel suggests that a reason why people choose the group change option is because individuals are rejected by the groups people wish to join.   This is particularly clear for black people in racist societies, for example.   Carers have had difficulty being accepted as having valued views in professional circles, although their willingness to engage in group action may be changing that. Meanwhile, users appear to continue to have difficulty in being accepted by such groups, although self-advocacy groups are being set up. They continue to be denied an option for change.

How useful is social identity theory? As a psychological theory about how individuals change their social situation it is most useful here as a measure of how far individuals have travelled in such change, as well as suggesting manifestos for action. Carers – at least the minority of carers who are 'politically' active – interviewed here appeared to have come some way in adopting the social route to individual empowerment. Workers also appear to be part of such a movement in a more undercover way, in their increasing role as advisers to carers in groups such as the QAGs. Users still have further to go. Meanwhile, managers are responding by reducing the value of the group, by not turning up or by rejecting their views.

There are some interesting comparisons to be made with the earlier discussion of Lukes' dimensions. Carers and managers were identified there as the more directly powerful groups, with workers showing their power more indirectly, and users consistently having the smallest amounts of power. In looking at Tajfel's theory as a theory of movements for change, the same power positions appear to be reinforcing themselves.

Chapter 4

Making empowerment real

In this chapter three areas will be concentrated on: firstly, the possible implications of this study for policy making; secondly, some analysis of the usefulness of the models presented here, including the analysis and development of existing community care policy and its impact on empowerment; and thirdly, the general use of theory.

Changing policy

In Chapter 1 it was argued that an incomplete model of human behaviour undermined grand models of organisations, because of a belief in 'rationalism' that did not in reality extend to such models of behaviour. In Chapter 2 it was argued that a bridge across the traditional divide between psychological theory and sociological and organisational theory could provide a more individual model of power and how it may be challenged. The argument was not merely about how we may analyse power but, to paraphrase Marx, also how individuals may change it.

The findings of this study reinforce the views expressed in Chapter 1 in suggesting that without positive and theoretically well-grounded ideas and methods of individual empowerment, organisational changes just reproduce traditional power relations.

The findings also highlight that a problem in achieving change is in how little agreement there is as to the meaning and practice of empowerment. The tendency in this study was for empowerment to be interpreted in a way that suited the stakeholder's own needs rather than following the explicit policy that community care was about empowering users. This shows how essential issues of power are to individuals, and it also suggests that a policy of empowerment can not be taken as read.

When such a policy was taken seriously there was little agreement as to what empowering users meant. Stakeholders produced their own differing analyses of what users wanted. If the quasi-market changes are about listening to users, then we may expect users' views of empowerment to dominate, but this does not appear to be happening. Rather, there appears to be an underlying message that the idea of users having a view on empowerment is still taboo as far as those in a position to do something about it are concerned.

Psychological and sociological theories, such as the ones used here, help in analysing such a situation, but they do not improve the power situation of users unless they are enabled to take advantage of the theoretical insights. While there is no agreement that this is appropriate or part of what is meant by a policy of empowerment, such enablement may not substantially happen.

Policy makers have adopted instead a top-down approach in dictating that certain groups are to be 'empowered'. But whatever the promise of a variety of political perspectives, the intended beneficiaries continue to be disempowered. If this is to change, there needs to be an understanding of how individuals are empowered and disempowered. This includes an understanding of the disempowering impact of decisions, whether meant positively or negatively, over which carers and users have no control.

How such an understanding can lead to empowerment without the active support of the powerful is also an essential question. But who are the powerful? Of those interviewed, this study suggests that carers and managers are the most directly powerful people in the lives of people with learning disabilities. There are likely to be many other actors who hold power who were not interviewed. The study reported the views of certain stakeholders of the perceived power of social services drivers. The impact of local and national politicians or their views on empowerment have not been explored. Managers in this study denied that they had much power, but an analysis of their words and actions led to a different conclusion. Politicians may have similar perceptions. The lack of recognition by the powerful of their power may be as great a problem as any deliberate disempowerment.

Useful theory

The faces of power

How useful have the theoretical positions been concerning the faces of power? There is strong evidence of the first and second 'faces of power', of direct influence and of issues being avoided and kept off the agenda. There is also some evidence of Lukes' third face, of people being forced to do what is not in their objective interests.

This study tends to show the variety of power 'vectors' rather than the clear presence of one dominating feature. With the first, and to a lesser extent, the second face of power, power can be seen as displayed by all participants. However, some features are more dominating than others, and these appear to reflect historical and traditional power positions (for instance, between professionals and carers, and carers and users). This is in line with Foucault's (1977) view of power as traditionally formed. His perception was also that those oppressed would react against such oppression, but he also suggested that such rebellion would easily become moulded along traditional power structures. That prediction appears to be reflected here as moves to user and carer involvement are shown by this study as also continuing to reflect historical power relations.

The message can be seen as 'the more things change, the more they stay the same', and a frustrating fatalism may be the result. The views of participants in this study were gathered in the context of organisational change. The findings appear to confirm the view, asserted in Chapter 1, that such change cannot empower without a deeper understanding of how people are empowered, and it challenges not only fatalism, but traditional power structures as well.

As a model, the four faces of power have enabled such an analysis, although information for such an analysis has come via the other two areas of theory as well. It is suggested that the sociological model is most effective when posed in the context of psychological and strategic models. This combination is also likely to be important in producing alternatives.

Theory and change

What proposals for change come from the four faces of power? Lukes' notion of three faces of power identifies power in terms of direct power relations, indirect power through systems organised to serve only specific powerful groups, and through people being forced by economic power relations to unconsciously act against their interests.

A response to this could be for power relations to be made more obvious and challengable, as far as the individual is concerned. The individual could be enabled to understand who has power and how it is used, and to understand how the power of others affects him/her, both directly and indirectly. An important issue is that the nature of Lukes' second and third faces means that they may be difficult to identify without support from others, as these do not involve directly observable power relations.

Foucault's ideas around the domination of historical and traditional forces suggests that we should challenge as well as identify power, but the nature of power means that it is also difficult for individuals to challenge. A key to a challenge may lie in this study's finding that all participants have some ability to apply power: a counter to Lukes' and

Foucault's tendency, criticised earlier, to see people as victims of other peoples' power.

Strategy

The findings here indicated frustration, fear and mistrust, with strategies of both exit and voice. They also suggest that reality is far more complicated than such analogies allow. However, the exit/voice/loyalty/neglect model has proven useful as a tool of analysis of the presence and use of the mechanisms of protest, complaint and alienation analogised by this model. In Chapter 1 the rationalism of organisational change was discussed and the implicit expectation of automatic use if people were given the opportunity to participate, complain, etc was questioned. In retrospect, the exit/voice/loyalty/neglect analogies are also based on such a rationalism. This study has identified the real human concerns that prevent such mechanisms being used in the rational way expected of them. It has also, perhaps, confirmed the criticisms made in Chapter 1 of mechanical organisational change models that dominate political science, and of the equally mechanical procedures that are based in such theory.

How does this theoretical area enable practice? The model of empowerment suggested here emphasises the awareness of, and the need to remove the causes of frustration, fear and mistrust in the use of procedures, rather than presuming a mechanical use. The exit/voice analogies suggest the ready availability of alternatives, such as choice in markets (exit), and use of the democratic process (voice). This study has suggested the difficulty in using, and lack of credibility of either. A practical proposition would be to attempt to change the reasons for such non-use and scepticism. This study has identified a fear of punishment by all participants, if protest or complaint is made, while choice is seen by users as not truly available. Managers should attempt to remove fear by encouraging protest and complaint, including direct funding of groups and workers to coordinate such protest, perhaps on the lines of community health councils, except more focused, more independent and more representative of carers and users.

With regard to the choice of resources, the community care changes put more power in the hands of managers and 'purchasing' social workers. The true test will be the extent to which this power is actually used on behalf of users and carers, or handed over to users and carers.

Psychology

Tajfel's social identity theory presents a model of individual development in a social world. It allows us to measure how far carers and users had come in asserting themselves and obtaining an increase in their self-value. Tajfel's analysis of social groups may also help analyse how to break down barriers that prevent individual entry to decision-making groups.

An assumption in the development of participation fora in social services departments appears to be that people will value taking part. However, carers may perceive only the stigma of such involvement where social services are seen negatively. A response has been to involve carers in reviewing the quality of services, through QAGs. In building such new 'ingroups' that overcome stigmatised perceptions, there is evidence from this study that users continue to be kept out, to be members of the 'outgroup' and objects of discrimination and exclusion. In Tajfel's analysis the presence of an outgroup helps keep the ingroup together. The successful involvement of carers may be to the further disadvantage of users.

Tajfel saw the bringing together of in- and outgroup members as crucial to overcoming mutual fear and stereotypes. Arguably CLDTs attempt to perform this role. They now seem threatened by the more individual approach of the quasi-market. To obtain a service, a carer or user must presently be willing to be seen as part of the stigmatised group that needs help from social services, rather than the use of social services improving the value of their social identity, as it may through a community approach that emphasises some say over the policy and rationing process. A key question from Tajfel's theory may be: how can social services operate so that involvement improves the individual's self-value within the quasi-market? Is this possible given restrictions on resources?

It is suggested that the psychological theories used here do actually enable a focus on individual needs. Social identity theory sees group membership as important to individual identity, and people making a choice between changing their group and moving to a new group where they are dissatisfied. This suggests that empowerment could be encouraged by enabling either road.

Looking at Tajfel's alternatives, workers can help improve the image of 'users' or 'carers' and help make their involvement in improving their situation a positive and meaningful experience. This may be through giving support to measures that build their confidence, such as QAG involvement.

It is difficult to distinguish between the notion of helping such a degree of group change and political involvement. Community work was discouraged in the early eighties as workers were accused of political involvement, in, for example, community development projects. Politicians who object to community work need to recognise that such political education is important. This will not be particularly easy, as it is likely that this will have an impact both on publicity (that may be seen as hostile by politicians), and on demands for resources.

It may be even more difficult to make possible individual change by improving access to membership of more powerful groups. The opening of doors by those powerful groups will be crucial, as will the campaigning of community care participants for those doors to be opened.

A conclusion that comes directly from Seligman's 'learned helplessness' theory and this study is the importance of control over your environment, of an approach to public services that allows such control, and positive encouragement to involvement in the planning and maintenance of resources. Abramson, Seligman and Teasdale (1978) identified a number of practical responses that came from Seligman's model and these were reported and extended earlier. These emphasise:

- the removal (or the reduction of the intensity) of negative outcomes through improving services and professional responses;

- the importance of controlling events through training and community development;

- the importance of an understanding that the reason for 'failure' may not be your fault but 'the system's' and political education may be a response.

Empowerment from theory

Figure 3 (p 63) summarises the above discussion and suggests some further possible empowerment responses. The following adds some of those ideas together as a test for a user and carer centred service or policy. Implicit in such a list is a belief in the value of carer and user as part of the policy-making process.

- Perceived control by participants. (Seligman)

- Perceived positive encouragement of users and carers. (Seligman)

- Perceived positive value, of the individual and of the social group of which the individual is a member, in their participation in the organisation. (Tajfel)

- Encouragement to use 'voice', whether through speaking out, complaining, standing for election, etc, and for this to be valued by managers and professionals. (exit/voice)

- Real and open access to choice. (exit/voice)
- Meetings to operate on the basis of open agendas, plain language and shared and equal membership. (Lukes and Tajfel)

- Power structures to be transparent. Hierarchies and decisions made at all levels should be open to view and to challenge. (Lukes and Seligman)

How does existing practice measure up? – the example of short-term care

In previous chapters there have been criticisms of the philosophy that lies behind the recent British community care policies. Doubt has been expressed as to whether such a philosophy is user-oriented despite the shared party political view that it is. The attempt in this section is to show how the above list, which shall be referred to as an 'audit structure', can help test whether we are now obtaining user-oriented services, and can support providers in developing such services.

The example of short-term care, or 'respite care' will be used here. This has been chosen because it was seen as a key area in the British white paper 'Caring for People'. In different forms it is a service that is provided for disabled adults and children by most social services departments (Young, 1988; Macadam and Robinson, 1995). It has been the subject of development internationally, with Sweden, USA and Australia enacting legislation to either enable short-term care or make it a legal right for disabled people (Wesway, 1995).

Short-term care has also been the subject of controversy:

> ... respite care is another term for crisis management, but it would not be necessary if disabled people received adequate and stable personal support .... While voluntary and unpaid personal assistants have to continue ... the need for respite care will increase and the position of the disabled person will continue to be both 'marginalised and invisible'. (Barnes, 1991, p 147)

Barnes and others have argued that short-term care meets carers' rather than users' needs. The Social Services Inspectorate (SSI) (1993) criticised the term 'respite care' for reinforcing this view.

Figure 3: Summary of theories and practical responses

Power theory	Interpretation	Suggested practical response
Sociological (eg, Lukes, Foucault)	■ Direct influence. ■ Systems organised to serve only traditional power groups; we may do things against our own interests but in the interests of those with power. ■ Historical and traditional forces dominate.	■ Understand who has power; understand how others' power affects you. ■ Make indirect and ideological power more obvious. ■ Challenge traditions of who has access to power.
Strategic exit/voice analogies	■ Choice or campaigning available to influence decision making. ■ Neglect as destructive and passive response.	■ Maximise possibilities in use of complaints processes and choice. ■ Maximise opportunities for protest. ■ Make access to choice and protest a positive not a fear-laden experience, eg, by removing possible punitive responses.
Social Identity Theory (eg, Tajfel)	■ Evaluative, cognitive and emotional interpretations of value of groups, which are important in personal identity. ■ Choice between individual and group approaches to empowerment.	■ Make joining groups a positive and meaningful experience. ■ Encourage group change through increasing confidence in joining groups, aided by community work. ■ Making possible individual change by making access to more powerful groups viable.
Learned Helplessness Theory (eg, Seligman)	■ Powerlessness due to consistent either negative or unpredictable responses to actions that leads to prediction of not being able to control environment.	■ Maximise opportunities for control. ■ Remove negative experiences of organisations by improving responses. ■ Make clear 'failure' may not be fault of individual but there are wider social processes that need changing.

It is suggested that the audit structure proposed here can help make the provision of short-term care more amenable to the needs of users. It cannot directly create the national policies that may need to change to give 'adequate and stable personal support'.

At the local level, where the purchaser/provider divide and contractual relationships increasingly dominate, an issue for service commissioners is what are appropriate and consistent contract conditions? How can comparisons be made between different forms of service as these develop? Short-term care may be with volunteer families, in residential care, through live-in carers and possibly a variety of other arrangements with little in common except 'care'. Which measures of quality are appropriate to all of these situations? This audit structure does not pretend to cover all aspects of quality but it does cover an important area that often may only be technically covered – the participation of the service user.

How do short-term care services match up with the audit structure suggested here?

Perceived control by participants

Who needs short-term care?

> A scheme of planned respite has proved a very attractive social workers option. Great efforts are made to arrange and book the residential home or substitute family .... Having gone through this painstaking process social workers may be surprised to discover the child does not actually go at the appointed time ... (the family) have been made to feel the answer is there, and they are wrong to take it .... (Middleton, 1992)

Research by Stalker and Robinson (1994) has reported stress by users, families and siblings while short-term care is provided. Middleton questions whether the short-term care used is always the choice of the user or the carer.

There appears to be some evidence that users and carers are not always in control either of the short-term care used or the process of choice. 'Control' has two aspects here. Most simply, users and carers could be offered genuine choices, and that issue will be addressed later. It is more essential for users and carers to have a say in the planning and provision of services. Questions may include the following:

- Which stakeholders were involved in the development of the service or in any subsequent changes?

- Which stakeholders are involved in the management of the service as a whole?

- Are carers and users involved in management or steering groups?

- Are there reviews? Who is involved in these and how?

- Is there a conscious or unconscious power structure within this involvement? If so, have attempts been made to equalise this structure? How? An example may be that users are only involved for part of a review and this reinforces existing power structures. Change would involve full participation, including opportunities for preparing for the review.

Perceived positive value

Family-based short-term care services are widely perceived by workers to be based on a partnership between participants. Is this perspective shared by all participants? Middleton and Barnes suggest that it is not. Which questions help identify a feeling of value among participants?

- In introducing users and carers to a short-term care resource, is care taken to ensure that any decision made reflects the views of the user? If such views are critical of part or all of the proposed placement, are there real attempts made to meet the issues raised?

- Is there subsequently a regular check made of the views of carers and users, and other stakeholders – through questionnaires, reviews and informal personal contact? Are the views that surface in these meetings channelled centrally and do they lead to change?

- If stakeholders are involved in planning and management, how far is this tokenist, or are the views of all stakeholders taken seriously, enabled and incorporated through changes in operation?

- What is the general attitude of workers and managers toward carers and users?

To an outsider, positive value may be indicated by the degree of sensitivity to user needs of the staff group, the amount of different forms of involvement, and how far the organisation has gone in taking on board the expressed views of stakeholders.

Encouragement to use voice

The Children Act 1989 and the community care legislation both talk of the involvement of users and carers in assessment for the provision of services. Research on the former (Macadam and Robinson, 1995) has suggested that this has only patchily been put into operation.

Important questions may be:

- How far do services go out of their way to encourage the presentation of views about the service?

- Do users and carers know who they can go to if they are not happy?

- Is it clear that there is encouragement and not sanctions towards those whose views are not in agreement with more powerful players – for instance, between users and carers?

- If there are differences between carers and users, how does the organisation go about resolving this – or are users' views ignored?

- Does the service have resources, including staff time, to use alternative communication tools, eg, where users have little or no spoken language, or have little knowledge of the language of committees?

- Is independent advocacy available?

- Are users encouraged to join self-advocacy groups?

- Are users and carers members of management groups and are they enabled to participate?

Real and open access to choice

Middleton (1992) has questioned whether carers and users have access to a choice of services. Rather, one form of short-term care may often be the only service offered.

There are some questions here for services:

- Are users and carers offered a choice in services?

- How far have they been involved in assessment for their needs that identified short-term care?

- Have they identified what they want?

- Have workers had their hands tied in offering only specific services?

- Have carers and users been told about the variety of short-term care services?

- Have they been enabled to review their choice?

The availability of a variety of different forms of short-term care may be a sign of success in this area.

Open agendas

Stress has been a reported finding of research into participants' views of short-term care. Maureen Oswin (1985) has reported the stress felt by parents who do not know which individuals will be looking after their children in residential short-term care.

Questions include:

- Many services already have long introductory periods that open up the information on users available to the service provider. Is this reciprocated through maximising the information about providers, which is made available to users?

- Do all stakeholders have equal access to information?

- Are users told detailed information about the resource they wish to use, or are they told very little?

- Are users involved throughout reviews and committees or only selected parts?

- Where there are meetings, how much help do stakeholders have in deciphering agendas?

- Do venues and times of meetings reflect all participants' needs, including physical access and any electronic aids?

The openness of agendas may be reflected by how understandable a local service is to an outside auditor.

Transparent power structures

Stress may be a reflection of the felt power position of carers and users.

Questions include:

- Do all stakeholders know about the agencies assessing for the service, and those providing it?

- Is it clear who has made the decisions about their eligibility for services, and who they can appeal to if they do not agree with official decisions?

- Do workers and managers understand the power structures of their organisations and are they able to use this knowledge to advise other stakeholders about how decisions are made, and how they can be challenged?

- Is the organisation open to be questioned about it's decisions?

- Do the most powerful members of the organisation go out of their way to consider the views and interests of users?

- Do complaints receive standard answers or has there been obvious consideration of the issues involved?
- How many stakeholders have tried but given up on presenting issues to the organisation, or do not feel confident in presenting a viewpoint?

Many of the above questions are not specific to the provision of short-term care. They are presented in the context of this essay as issues that come out of the structures that now exist for care services following the NHS and Community Care Act 1990. The proposition here is that we can not depend on this legislation, despite the political assertions surrounding it, to automatically empower users. Rather, we need detailed methods of enabling and checking services for empowerment.

Analysing policy

The audit approach presented here may also be usable in looking at broad policy areas. Figure 4 (p 69) makes a first and incomplete attempt to use the above approaches to look at the two community care approaches that were discussed in Chapter 1: decentralisation and the new quasi-market. Using Figure 4, neither approach fully meets the requirements identified by the author as important to empowerment.

There are positives and negatives in each area. Eligibility and rationing are key issues. For those eligible to enter the state care market, there is some control through choice, encouragement and a reinforcement of a feeling of value through involvement in the assessment process. There are also transparent power relations, through contracts.

For those who have not cleared the assessment hurdle, or feel unable to approach this hurdle, such control, feeling of value and encouragement do not exist. Meanwhile, the power relations that construct the hurdles are frequently not clear, particularly with the health service, where quangos do not have the accessibility of councillors, although even here this study has suggested suspicion as to the councillor's role.

There are similar issues with decentralisation. The notion of a local service suggests a more controllable service with encouragement to use the service, involvement valued, meetings with open agendas, and clear power structures through users and carers knowing those with power. This study has suggested the reality is often perceived differently with users having little choice, and frequently this is perceived as at the whim of workers. Even with meetings, such as QAGs, where carers and users are encouraged to give their views, these were seen as obstructed by the indifference of senior managers.

Figure 4: Services compared: using the issues identified in this
study

	Decentralised service	Market changes
Perceived control by participants	+ve: local service. Contact with workers. -ve: no rights to service. Little choice.	+ve: access to choice. -ve: no rights to service. Choice only if eligible. Narrowness of eligibility.
Positive encouragement	+ve: community work by CLDTs. -ve: workers selective.	+ve: implicit involvement in assessment process. -ve: hurdles before assessed and in obtaining service.
Value of participation	+ve: encouragement by local workers. -ve: discouragement in committees, etc.	+ve: encouragement if eligible. -ve: discouragement if ineligible.
Use of voice	+ve: QAGs, some policy changes. -ve: seen as challenging "vociferous minority".	+ve: getting higher up eligibility list? Rights of complaint, etc. -ve: no substantive rights.
Choice	+ve: know more from local CLDTs, what choices are. -ve: limited to what exists. Users at whim of workers.	+ve: choice to those eligible. -ve: access to choice limited.
Open agendas	+ve: QAGs becoming equal. Workers more subject to criticism by carers. -ve: limited to participators. Managers do not go to QAG. Other meetings not open.	+ve: clear contracting arrangements. -ve: tendency to quangoisation in quasi-markets.

There are contradictions between the basic organisational structures that are needed to empower, through enabling control and participation, and systems meant to debar entry as part of an organisation's operation.   Work still needs to be done on how organisations can both ration and empower.

Using theory

This study used three theoretical perspectives as a framework to look at power.   It is suggested here that they have helped form a fairly comprehensive analysis of the power position of people with learning disabilities, their carers, professionals and managers in one borough.

At the start of Chapter 2 the author insisted that he was not building an immutable grand plan, rather he spoke of a 'set of analogies'. A framework was presented, built on definitions of power, strategies of power, and psychological analyses.   The three distinct analyses were used in a unified way that has helped comprehend personal power positions and their interlinkages in terms of one set of public services.   It is not being suggested that the particular theoretical assertions used are the only possible positions.   The three areas of theory – psychology, the strategic and the structural – may be what is important.   Crespi (1992) has also analysed power in terms of three dimensions – the inner subjective (the psychological), the outer subjective (the social psychological) and the objective/structural (the sociological) – primarily using psychodynamic theory.

Foucault (1979b) pointed to the work of Machiavelli in showing how power strategies are formed and are used at a local level.   Clegg (1989) attempted to bring together Machiavellian and traditional Hobbesian rationalist dominant power theses together in terms of non-monolithic distinct 'circuits of power', although these do not appear to include an explicit psychological dimension.   The practical use of such theories has been shown as possible here.   It is suggested that the next steps should be to:

- use the same theoretical perspectives to analyse other interrelationships or organisations;

- use other psychological and strategic theories in similar analyses;

- to use such analyses to support users in understanding the basis of their own disempowerment and future empowerment.

References

Abramson, L., Seligman, M. and Teasdale, J. (1978) 'Learned helplessness in humans: critique and reformulation', *Journal of Abnormal Psychology*, vol 87, no 1, pp 49-74.

Atherton, C. (1989) 'The welfare state: still on solid ground?', *Social Service Review*, 63, pp 167-79.

Audit Commission (1992a) Community care: managing the cascade of change, London: HMSO.

Audit Commission (1992b) The community revolution: personal social services and community care, London: HMSO.

Bachrach, P. and Baratz, M.S. (1970) Power and poverty, Oxford: Oxford University Press.

Barnes, C. (1991) Disabled people in Britain and discrimination, London: Hurst and Co.

Barry, N. (1990) 'Markets, citizenship and the welfare state: some critical reflections', in R. Plant and N. Barry, *Citizenship and rights in Thatcher's Britain: two views*, London: IEA Health and Welfare Unit.

Beresford, P. and Croft, S. (1986) Whose welfare?, Brighton: Lewis Cohen Urban Studies Centre.

Bradshaw, J. (1972) 'The taxonomy of social need', New Society 19, p 496.

Brown, H. and Smith, H. (1992) Normalisation: a reader for the nineties, London: Routledge.

Brown, S. and Wistow, G. (1990) The roles and tasks of community mental handicap teams, Aldershot: Avebury/CRSP.

Buchanan, J.M. et al (1978) The economics of politics, London: IEA.

Challis, L. (1990) Organising public services, Harlow: Longman.

Clegg, S. (1989) Frameworks of power, London: Sage.

Crespi, F. (1992) Social action and power, Oxford: Blackwell.

Dalley, G. (1988) Ideologies of caring, Basingstoke: Macmillan.

Dalley, G. (1992) 'Social welfare ideologies and normalisation: links and conflicts', in H. Brown and H. Smith, *Normalisation: a reader for the nineties*, London: Routledge.

Digeser, P. (1992) 'The fourth face of power', *Journal of Politics*, vol 54, no 4, pp 977-1007.

Doyal L. and Gough, I. (1991) *A theory of human need*, Basingstoke: Macmillan.

Foucault, M. (1979a) *Discipline and punish*, Harmondsworth: Penguin.

Foucault, M. (1979b) *Politics and reason*, reprinted in M. Foucault, *Politics, philosophy, culture: interviews and other writings 1977-1984*, New York: Routledge, Chapman and Hall.

Foucault, M. (1983) *Critical theory/intellectual history*, reprinted in M. Foucault, *Politics, philosophy, culture: interviews and other writings 1977-1984*, New York: Routledge, Chapman and Hall.

Foucault, M. (1984) *On power*, reprinted in M. Foucault, *Politics, philosophy, culture: interviews and other writings 1977-1984*, New York: Routledge, Chapman and Hall.

Foucault, M. (1988) *Politics, philosophy, culture: interviews and other writings 1977-1984*, New York: Routledge, Chapman and Hall.

Graham, H. (1983) 'Caring: a labour of love', in J. Finch and D. Groves (eds), *A labour of love: women, work and caring*, London: Routledge Kegan Paul.

Hambleton, R. (1988) 'Consumerism, decentralisation and local democracy', *Public Administration*, vol 66, pp 125-47.

Hambleton, R. and Hoggett, P. (1990) *Beyond excellence: quality local government in the 1990s*, Bristol: SAUS Publications, Working Paper 85.

Harré, R. (1993) *Social being*, 2nd edn, Oxford: Blackwell.

Hewstone, M. and Antaki, C. (1988) 'Attribution theory and social explanations', in M. Hewstone, W. Stroebe, et al, *Introduction to social psychology*, Oxford: Blackwell.

Hirschman, A. (1970) *Exit, voice and loyalty: responses to decline in firms, organisations and states*, Cambridge, Mass.: Harvard University Press.

Hodgwood, B. and Gunn, L. (1984) *Policy analysis in the real world*, Oxford: Oxford University Press.

Kitzinger, C. (1991) 'Feminism, psychology and the paradox of power', *Feminism and Psychology*, vol 1 (1), pp 111-29.

LeGrand, J. (1990) *Quasi-markets and social policy*, Bristol: SAUS Publications.

Lukes, S. (1974) *Power: a radical view*, Basingstoke: Macmillan.

Lyons, W.E. and Lowery, D. (1986) 'The organisation of political space: citizen responses to dissatisfaction in urban communities', *Journal of Politics,* vol 48, pp 321-46.

Macadam, R. and Robinson, C. (1995) *Balancing the Act: the affect of the Children Act on family link services,* London: NCB.

Middleton, L. (1992) *Children first,* Venture Press.

Neville, R. (1995) *Hippie, hippie shake,* London: Bloomsbury.

NSPCC (1994) *ABCD training pack,* Leicester: NSPCC.

Niskanen, W.A. (1973) *Bureaucracy: servant or master?,* London: IEA.

Oliver, M. (1990) *The politics of disablement,* Basingstoke: Macmillan.

Oswin, M. (1985) *They keep going away,* London: King's Fund Centre.

Pascale, R. (1990) *Managing on the edge,* Harmondsworth: Penguin.

Peterson, C. and Seligman, M. (1984) 'Causal explanations as a risk factor for depression: theory and evidence', *Psychological Review,* vol 91, no 3, pp 347-74.

Plant, R. and Barry, N. (1990) *Citizenship and rights in Thatcher's Britain: two views,* London: IEA Health and Welfare Unit.

Rees, S. (1991) *Achieving power: practice and policy in social welfare,* Sydney: Allen and Unwin.

Rose, H. (1994) *Love, power and knowledge,* Cambridge, UK: Polity Press.

Seligman, M.E.P. (1975) *Helplessness,* San Francisco: W.H. Freeman.

Social Services Inspectorate (1993) *Guidance on standards for short-term breaks,* London: HMSO.

Smith, H. and Brown, H. (1992) 'Inside-out: a psychodynamic approach to normalisation', in H. Brown and H. Smith, *Normalisation: a reader for the nineties,* London: Routledge.

Sogyal Rinpoche (1992) *The Tibetan book of living and dying,* London: Rider Books.

Stalker, K. and Robinson, C. (1994) 'Parents' view of different respite care services', *Mental Handicap Research,* 7(2), pp 97-117.

Tajfel, H. (1981) *Human groups and social categories: studies in social psychology,* Cambridge: Cambridge University Press.

Taylor, M., Hoyes, L., Lart, R. and Means, R. (1992) *User empowerment in community care: unravelling the issues,* Bristol: SAUS Publications.

Tyne, A. (1982) 'Community care and mentally handicapped people', in A. Walker (ed.) *Community care: the family, the state and social policy,* Oxford: Basil Blackwell and Martin Robertson.

Taylor-Goodby, P. (1991) *Social change, social welfare and social science*, Hemel Hempstead: Harvester Wheatsheaf.

Ungerson, C. (1987) *Policy is personal: sex, gender and informal care*, London: Tavistock.

Wesway, (1995) *Rendezvous on respite*: international conference, March 1995, Thunder Bay: Wesway.

Wolfensberger, W. (1980) 'The definition of normalisation: update, problems, disagreements, and misunderstandings', in R.J. Flynn and K.E. Nitsch, *Normalisation, social integration and community services*, Baltimore: Baltimore University Press.

Young, P. (1988) *The provision of care in supported lodgings and unregistered homes*, London: OPCS.

Appendix

Interview structure

Front-line workers, carers and managers

I have chosen people to interview on the basis of their historical knowledge of the service for people with learning disabilities in Dudley. However, the study is not particularly about Dudley, but about your and others views of power and empowerment and the experience of these by workers, managers and carers and users. That means I will be asking you for some of your history of Dudley's services for people with learning disabilities.

1. (Based on direct and indirect power)

What influence and authority do you believe (1) managers; (2) front-line workers; (3) carers; (4) users have on the lives of people with learning disabilities?

Looking back at the history of the services, do you think there have been changes in how such authority has been used? Can you give examples of how the statutory authorities have used their authority, first from when you started work in Dudley and more recently?

Do you believe that this has generally been influence in terms of power over or power in support of users and carers? Can you give examples if either? Has this changed over the period of time you have worked for Dudley?

In what ways have national and local policies had an impact on the power/influence/authority workers and managers have over, and in support of users and carers? Again, can you give examples of practice following different policy changes, eg, following introduction of CLDTs and likely impact of community care changes?

Do you believe such influence has been beneficial? How? How not?

Are there underlying problems that prevent such influence always being used on behalf of carers and users? What are these?

Where do you think power lies in services for people with learning disabilities?

2. Strategy (from exit/voice)

What official avenues are there for carers and users to express their needs and views? Can you give a description of how these have been positively used? What alternatives might there be?

What avenues are available for carers and users if they do not, for example, like a service that has been offered, or how it has been offered? Can you give an example of a dissatisfied client, both recently and earlier on in your career?

Are there possibilities for carers and users to campaign for better resources, for example? Can you give examples both now and in the past about when this has happened and what the impact and response of the statutory authorities was?

What rights do you see carers and users having within Dudley?

How meaningful are official platforms, eg, complaints procedures?

What happens to complaints, questions, comments?

3. (from psychology theories)

(Helplessness)

How often has carers' and users' participation in either their own reviews, etc, or in consultation procedures led to real change?

Can you give some descriptions of what happened?

Have there been carers and users who have dropped out of service planning? Why do you think this has happened?

Why don't more people participate actively in planning services, in your view?

What steps have been taken to improve involvement?

What do you think could happen?

With the steps that have been taken, is it carers' and users' fault if they do not benefit from the support of statutory authorities?

(Social Identity Theory)

Can individual carers and users affect change, either in their 'case' or in terms of policy? Can you give examples of this?

Is it realistic to expect carers and users to affect change? Why/why not?

Are carer and user participants considered by other participants as having the same value as the professionals?

Is change more likely to be achieved by carers and users in groups or as individuals? Can you give examples of this? Has this improved the view of professionals of the value of carers and users?

Do individuals readily join groups to improve their lot? If not, why is that?

Questions to users

1. Can you give me your story about how you ended up living here/ how you get on at the centre? Did you have a choice about when you went?

I am particularly interested in people such as social workers, community nurses, people who work at the centre, etc. Have they been helpful to you? Can you say how? Have they tended to tell you what to do? Would you rather they did not? Do you think there is really a job for such people to do?

Do you think people like social workers are always able to help you in the ways you would like? What do you think stops them?

2. If you had a complaint, what would you do? Who would you take it to? Have you ever done this or know someone else who did? Can you tell me about it? Do you know what would happen to the complaint?

If there has been a problem at centres or places you have lived at have you found it easy to say anything or make yourself understood? What happened?

Have you ever got together with other people to try and get something new at the centre? What happened?

3. Can you tell me about meetings you go to at the centres or at home? When you have been to those meetings, do you think you are treated as seriously as other people there? Who do you think is treated more seriously than you? Do you want to go regularly? Why? Who has no say, and why?

Do you think you have helped change things for yourself or everybody by having your say?